Palgrave Studies in Literature, Science and Medicine

Series Editors

Sharon Ruston, Department of English and Creative Writing, Lancaster University, Lancaster, UK

Alice Jenkins, School of Critical Studies, University of Glasgow, Glasgow, UK

Jessica Howell, Department of English, Texas A&M University, College Station, USA

Palgrave Studies in Literature, Science and Medicine is an exciting, prize-winning series that focuses on one of the most vibrant and inter-disciplinary areas in literary studies: the intersection of literature, science and medicine. Comprised of academic monographs, essay collections, and Palgrave Pivot books, the series will emphasize a historical approach to its subjects, in conjunction with a range of other theoretical approaches. The series will cover all aspects of this rich and varied field and is open to new and emerging topics as well as established ones.

Vincent Bruyere

Epidemiological Realism

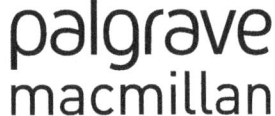

Vincent Bruyere
Department of French and Italian
Emory University
Atlanta, GA, USA

ISSN 2634-6435   ISSN 2634-6443 (electronic)
Palgrave Studies in Literature, Science and Medicine
ISBN 978-3-031-68516-3   ISBN 978-3-031-68517-0   (eBook)
https://doi.org/10.1007/978-3-031-68517-0

This Palgrave Macmillan imprint is published by the registered company Springer Nature
Switzerland AG
The registered company address is: Gewerbestrasse 11, 6330 Cham, Switzerland

If disposing of this product, please recycle the paper.

Acknowledgments

This book was a long time in the making but its argument really started to take shape in 2021, thanks to a series of seminars and talks at the University of Warwick, George Washington University, Dartmouth College Institute of French Cultural Studies, and the French Consulate in Atlanta. I would like to thank Oliver Davis, Pauline Goul, Larry Kritzman, and Louise Shaw for their invitations to think about public health from a humanistic perspective. As curator of the David J. Sencer CDC Museum, Louise gave me a unique opportunity to peak behind the scenes. I am most grateful for her invitation to join the board of the *Influenza* exhibit in 2019, where I learned a great deal about what it means to gather stories and objects pertaining to public health. I am also very grateful for the collegiality and hospitality of the Center for Apocalyptic and Post-Apocalyptic Studies (CAPAS) at the University of Heidelberg where I had the good fortune of spending a semester in 2023. The vignettes on mold horror and fungal anxiety greatly benefitted from conversations with the members of the working group on apocalyptic affects (Katie Barclay, Jana Cattien, Jenny Stümer, and Susan Watkins). At Emory, I can always count on the support of the chair of the French and Italian department, Valérie Loichot, and all my colleagues. Many ideas were generated in conversation with pre-med, pre-health, and pre-nursing students who are now healthcare professionals or working toward that goal. I am indebted to their presence in the classroom, their open-mindedness, and their commitment to learning. At Palgrave, I would like to thank Molly Beck for taking a chance on a rather untraditional project and the editors of Palgrave Studies in Literature, Science and Medicine for welcoming the book in their series. I would also like to thank Timothy Campbell for his encouragements at a time where I needed them. Finally, I want to acknowledge the emotional support and the sense of respite I have received from my family on both sides of the Atlantic, and above all, on the home front, day in day out, rain or shine, from my husband, Aaron. Goodnight Sumter.

Competing Interests The authors have no conflicts of interest to declare.

CONTENTS

LIST OF FIGURES

CHAPTER 1

Stinky Contexts (Abbott Pandemic Defense Coalition 2023)

Abstract There is such a thing as epidemiological realism because epidemiological concepts and concerns have seeped into the fabric of social life, redrawing in the process the contours of the body, while shifting a shared sense of ordinariness. Terms like "exposure," "contamination," "PCR," "risk," "confinement," "droplets," "variants," "PPE," "herd immunity," "fomites" have people talking, taking sides, telling stories, and listening intently in a state of heightened receptivity to anecdotal evidence, contested models, and debunked theories. As such, epidemiological realism inevitably brings into focus issues of shared competency between domains of expertise. The point of this book, however, is not to recover what epidemiologists already know (about rabies, about HIV/AIDS, about Alzheimer) in an incidental archive made up of stories people tell (about rabies, HIV/AIDS, or Alzheimer). It is to meet halfway the world of chance encounters between humans, animals, and infrastructures in which epidemiology deploys its repertoire of gestures and concepts.

Keywords Berlant, Lauren · Epidemiology · Realism · Ordinariness · Testing · Wastewater

© The Author(s), under exclusive license to Springer Nature Switzerland AG 2024
V. Bruyere, *Epidemiological Realism*, Palgrave Studies in Literature, Science and Medicine,
https://doi.org/10.1007/978-3-031-68517-0_1

In a short video released by the Abbott Pandemic Defense Coalition in 2023, a researcher explains that "wastewater shows what passes through people, things people are infected with, things that are on people's skin. Anything that gets washed down the drain [...]" adding emphatically— as if to elevate the humbling gesture—"Can you believe that 50 mill sample that you took represents a whole community?" In this book, I take that question at heart, not necessarily to cultivate disbelief in the kind of collective representations public health deploys in the world and the kind of affective spell this deployment casts on a population, but rather to attend to the worldbuilding properties of epidemiology through the lens of critical theory, literary analysis, and visual culture.

A "world" is being summoned by wastewater surveillance in the sense that Erich Auerbach talks about the world of Homer and the world of the Hebrew Bible with the understanding that Homer's world and the world of the Hebrew Bible are not the same. In the world where Euryclea recognizes the scar on Odysseus while washing a stranger's feet, "nothing must remain hidden and unexpressed" (Auerbach 2013), whereas the world where Abraham binds Isaac leaves room to the unexpressed, bringing certain parts into high relief and leaving others into obscurity.[1] In the world of wastewater surveillance, pandemics occur as the ransom of collective life, reality is accessed from the vantage of critical orifices, and we shed cells together. A "we" exists in connection with a sewage system and a somewhat odious truth telling exercise—let's have a look at what you flush and I'll tell you how you belong[2] (Figs. 1.1 and 1.2).

The Abbott Pandemic Defense Coalition vignette seeks to occupy the perceptual field that epidemiology defined a century earlier around the story of Dr. John Snow and the Broad Street water pump during the 1854 cholera epidemic in London. Much has been written about the legendary status of Snow's map with its cluster of cases conveniently pointing at the source of transmission. More saliently, Sari Altschuler (2021, 140–144) has pressed against the seductive promises of mastery in matters of public health at work in its retelling: the time has come to tell a different

---

[1] On the notion of world in Auerbach see Hayot (2011, 142).

[2] It bears noting with Jonathan Strauss that in the novels of Victor Hugo the sewer is already "a place of memory, a reservoir that holds the lost consciousness of the city and that remembers, in a material, degraded, but somehow more authentic form, the ancient turmoil of those above" (2012, 249).

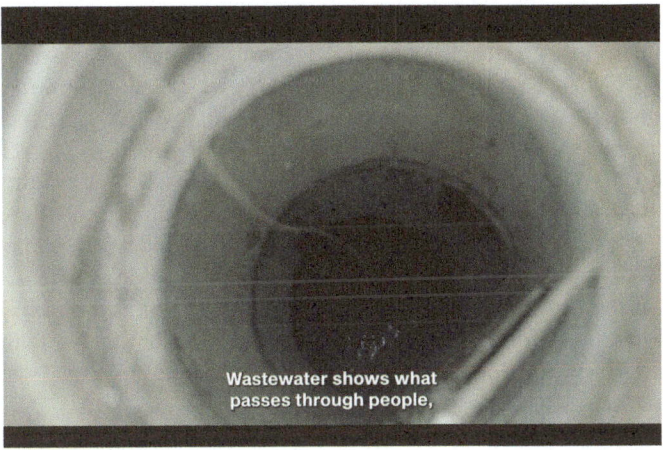

Fig. 1.1 Wastewater surveillance. "The Virus Hunt: USA." Abbott Pandemic Defense Coalition, 2023. https://www.youtube.com/watch?v=t686Kibr1-A

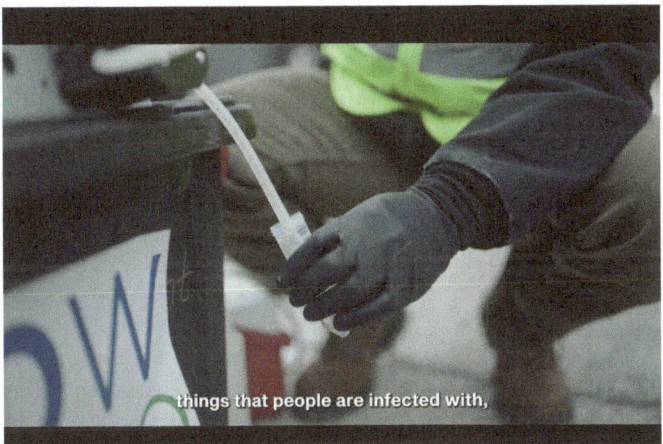

Fig. 1.2 Wastewater surveillance. "The Virus Hunt: USA." Abbott Pandemic Defense Coalition, 2023. https://www.youtube.com/watch?v=t686Kibr1-A

origin story that doesn't rely on the fantasy of dissociating the problem at hand from its infrastructure. Wastewater surveillance too is doing some dissociative work. The equation between dirty water and community is at once extraordinary and yet the images attached to it are unremarkable. The sample promises representation and gives us nothing to see. There is what a group of experts invests in a sensing device and there is, implicitly, the story being told about depth and flatness, above ground privacy and the underground commons. The gloved hands that collect the sample and tuck it away hold on to its groundbreaking representational promise while the rest of the vignette tries to ground the legibility it seeks to publicize in a spatial configuration that needs to retain enough elements of familiarity (the Chicago skyline and headless silhouettes walking on a busy street) to remain relatable.

What I hope this peculiar point of entry into my argument will convey—even if it is at the cost of courting a rather repulsive realm— is a sense that there is more to epidemiology than the "study of the distribution and determinants of health-related states among specified populations and the application of that study to the control of health problems"(CDC Public Health 101 2024). Epidemiology also registers relations and possibilities "that have not been registered before"—to echo Fredric Jameson's minimalist definition of realism (2010, 362. See also 2015, 146). Historically, literary realism has functioned as an answer to the question of how narrative creatures are supposed to occupy the middle-distance between the inertia of the landscape in the background and the stillness of the objects within reach. Today realism is the term around which literary theory and cultural studies tend to congregate when debating the ordinariness of the world and how much accidental predictability the world can take.[3] The idea of epidemiological realism seeks to relocate that debate outside the confines of a conversation where the borders of realism are other "isms" (naturalism, modernism, romanticism, postmodernism). The point is not to dismiss the validity of these "-isms" and their capacity to draw narrative objects together or to draw

---

[3] In the preface-manifesto to *Pierre et Jean*, Guy Maupassant writes: "The number of persons on earth who die every day in an accident is considerable. But can we drop a tile, or through her under the wheels of a car in the middle of a story, under the pretext that accidents happen?" (1888, xvi–xvii). See also Gosh: "Probability and the modern novel are in fact twins, born at about the same time, among the same people, under a shared star that destined the, to work as vessels for the containment of the same kind of experience" (2016, 16).

boundaries between them and their outlook on the world they care to summon. Rather it is to reframe what it means to put literary and cultural studies to work in the epidemiological present. It is to add more borders, to create more segments, more sequences, and introduce new sequencing logics with more overlaps and folding lines in an attempt to substantiate the claim that, whether we want it or not, we live in an epidemiological reality.

Lauren Berlant explains that "any object/scene could come to belong to a realist genre—an anecdote, an uncanny sound, a dream, a pet, or a cookie. What matters is the presence of a relation that invests an object/scene with the prospects of the world's continuity" (2011, 52). The realism they have in mind here is not necessarily the one that literary historians locate in a timeline and oppose to modernism and romanticism. It is a form of emotional expertise about the world one is stuck with. Likewise, epidemiological realism is not readily available as a fully formed object of inquiry awaiting an authoritative description. It describes a form of emotional expertise about a world of chance encounters between incidence and coincidence, populations and infrastructures, between "the wrong bat" and "the wrong pig"—to echo the tagline of Steven Soderbergh epidemiological thriller, *Contagion* (2011), to which I will return later in the book. If literary realism is about the ordinary and extraordinary dramas of a world where characters A, B, C, and D do not have to meet or be acquainted with each other to belong to the name narrative universe (Anderson 2006, 25), epidemiological realism tells us the stories of a world where "A [is] sick while B, at his elbow, stayed well, but C, at B's elbow, fell sick of A's disease" (Geddes Smith cited in Wald 2008, 21).

Epidemiological realism tends to be statistical (as in projection modeling and risk management) or proxemic (as in contact tracing and outbreak narratives) but it doesn't have to be. An anecdote, a diagram, a concept, an image, a tedious formality, even a turbid sample can too become sites of forecasting and the loci of one's membership in a population, or for that matter, a source of existential puzzlement.[4] It is that range of possibilities that this book is after and pursues through a series of

---

[4] Barbara Duden describes such a scene of puzzlement in her work on the representation of the unborn: "The counselor pointed out the curve on a diagram that showed the statistical risk of malformed children for New York mothers older than thirty-five. Did Maria grasp that her age was being made into an issue? I could see that the graph left

vignettes in which epidemiological concepts and concerns are at play but do not saturate scenes of reluctant belonging and contagious commonalities, thus leaving enough room for other interpretive maneuvers to flourish in their midst.

Epidemiological Realism joins a chorus of recent interventions situated on the border between public health, global health, disease ecology, epidemiology, and humanistic inquiry. Christos Lynteris's anthropological readings of pestilence narratives and figures and Allison Kenner's urban ethnography of bodies out of breath understand the epidemiology of zoonoses and chronic illnesses as a site of inquiry into the Anthropocenic collapse of categorical distinctions between natural, political, immunological, literary, local, and global histories. In *Avian Reservoirs*, Frédéric Keck has shown how the distinctions between nature and culture relayed by anthropologists to study human societies and their others (gods and animals, animal-gods) shift or sway in response to zoonotic events or in preparation for their eventuality. With *Epidemiological Realism*, I too seek to occupy these scenes and sites of collapse but from a literary and aesthetic perspective that is often missing in the conversation. To do so, I insist on the ordinariness of epidemiology.

If there is such a thing as epidemiological realism, it is because epidemiological concepts and concerns have seeped into the fabric of social life, redrawing the contours of the body (does it end with the skin and at one's fingertips, or with the air it breathes in and out and the cells it sheds?) in the process, while shifting a shared sense of ordinariness and flexing contrarian muscles. Terms like "exposure," "contamination," "PCR," "risk," "confinement," "droplets," "variants," "PPE," "herd immunity," "fomites" have people talking, taking sides, telling stories, and listening intently in a state of heightened receptivity to anecdotal evidence, contested models, and debunked theories. As such, epidemiological realism inevitably brings into focus issues of shared competency between domains of expertise. In this version of interdisciplinarity, however, the point is not to recover what epidemiology already knows about rabies, about HIV/AIDS, about Alzheimer in an incidental archive made up of stories people tell about rabies, HIV/AIDS, or Alzheimer. I am more interested in what it means for epidemiology to come to bear on rituals of meaning making in the humanities. In other

her confused. [...] The counselor's insistence on risk made little sense to [her]" (1993, 27–27).

words, I posit the ordinariness of epidemiology to better understand what a training in literary criticism and the history of representation could possibly have to say about the challenge of inhabiting critically the stinky contexts opened up by sensing devices and public health campaigns.[5]

Of course, these days nobody needs to be reminded of public health and of the reach of epidemiology in our lives. The concept of epidemiological realism is yet another moving part in an ongoing conversation on the contours of the COVID-19 present. Like Benjamin Bratton, I ask, "What are the form of 'the real' that the pandemic has forced us to confront?" (2021, 3) but I follow a rather different path. Bratton's argument is driven by a polemical diagnosis of the failure of political philosophy valuing an aesthetic of resistance to respond to the COVID societal challenge other than as a technophobic critique of surveillance—more on that in the concluding vignette. Mine is an impersonal post-confinement diary organized around the close reading of a broad range objects and stories from the recent and not so recent past: films and music videos, photography, poetry, paintings and engravings from the early modern period, contemporary illness narratives, and a sixteenth-century chronicle commemorating a rabies outbreak in a rural area in Eastern France.

At Emory University in Atlanta, where, among other things I teach literature, the main campus of the Centers for Disease Control and Prevention (CDC) is always in the background. It is the view from my office. The isolation unit where Ebola patients were treated in 2014 is around the corner, surrounded by the schools of public health and the school of nursing, and the school medicine. The lay of the land, the colleagues I get to meet, the students I get to work with, and the conversations I can't help but overhear in the bus have serendipitous ways to remind me I live in an epidemiological reality. After all this is what literary scholars tend to do. They keep watch. They join overheard conversations

---

[5] The idea of stinky context is inspired by the mischievous title of Rita Felski, "Context Stinks!" (2011). "Context Stinks!", she explains, is a double quotation from Bruno Latour in *Reassembling the Social* (2005) citing starchitect Rem Koolhaas. The rejoinder is meant as a provocation to widen the range of interpretive dynamics scholars typically cultivate to index the meaning of artworks but also raise the stakes of interpretive works, which is very much in line with my ambitions. There is no reason why, Felski argues, criticism endgame should be to explain texts away rather than describe them as forms of attachments with a certain agency. In that spirit, *Epidemiological Realism* considers objects and stories as affective and aesthetic nodes in the interconnected states described by epidemiology.

in an effort "to make the literary object of study [...] more connected with what goes on in a blatantly political world" (Hartman 1995, 543). But how are literary studies supposed to catch up with what's going on in a blatantly epidemiological world? That is, in a world where, precisely, epidemiological concepts are making their way in the repertoire of forms and tropes that people rely on to make sense of intimacy, plan out what it is reasonable to hope, reinvent rituals, let go of a certain sense of freedom, and magnetize frustration and loss of agency. *Epidemiological Realism* is a version of that serendipity.

CHAPTER 2

Epidemiological Realism (*The Horla* 1887)

Abstract My argument is driven by an initial set of propositions that I locate in an early fable of pandemic extinction written by Guy de Maupassant in 1887. Proposition 1: Epidemiological realism is not about how realistic representations of epidemic events are. It is about the planetarity of a world governed by epidemiological principles that apply everywhere and explain everything that falls within their purview. Proposition 2 and 3 correspond to the operational frame within which security experts anticipating on the next pandemic crisis and its impact on political institutions and social infrastructures learn from scenario-based exercises. It means that epidemiological events are not immediately available to us as objects of inquiry and concern but only through the lens of narrative and visual conventions that either substantiate or deflate the claims to crisis. Proposition 4: Epidemiological realism lends expression to forms of hyperawareness that at time can be difficult to bear. It registers and assesses disturbances in the conventions of relating random misfortunes to systemic affliction, and vice versa.

Keywords Collective psychosis · Extinction · Fiction · Horla · Maupassant, Guy · Pandemic · Preparedness

© The Author(s), under exclusive license to Springer Nature Switzerland AG 2024
V. Bruyere, *Epidemiological Realism*, Palgrave Studies in Literature, Science and Medicine,
https://doi.org/10.1007/978-3-031-68517-0_2

My argument is not driven by a chronology but an initial set of propositions that I locate in an early fable of pandemic extinction written by Guy de Maupassant. In *The Horla* (1887)—or "The Entity" in Joachim Neugroschel translation (2003)—the horizon of contagion is colonial, planetary, and world-ending but it is also ordinary and indexed the realist production of bourgeois daily life. In this configuration, realism is at once a system of beliefs in something tangibly new and immediate and a training in these beliefs.[1] Maupassant's narrator wants nothing more than to believe that he wants the world he inhabits and the way things in it come together and fall neatly into place for people like him. He lives in the ruins of the hierarchical structures that once held the *ancien régime* together and clings to the remnants of the old order, to a terroir, to genealogy, to the tree that grows in front of his mansion, and to the root metaphor. At the same time, he is responsive and even attuned to the pull of the present and the lure of what's out there, as evidenced by the diary he keeps over a five-month period, whose entries add up to compose the story we read.

What's most remarkable about "The Horla" from the vantage of epidemiological realism is the fact that the production of daily life lodges itself in what is essentially an epidemiological plot responding to a disturbance in the fabric of someone's sense of ordinariness. The disturbance is affective at first. It is only a feeling, a mix of fear, restlessness, and anxiety. Then, as the malaise worsens, the feeling becomes symptomatic in the form of inexplicable cravings, bodies that waste away in the absence of conclusive diagnosis, night terrors, even negative hallucinations, and a loss of agency, as if something or someone else had taken control of one's will. The diarist conducts experiments and gathers evidence to determine

---

[1] See Jameson, 1985. Here Jameson's go-to text is Gustave Flaubert's novella, *A Simple Heart* [1877], in part because it had already been Roland Barthes's go-to text in a landmark essay on the production of bourgeois reality (1968). It bears noticing that "The Horla" and *A Simple Heart* are not entirely unrelated: Maupassant was Flaubert protégé. André Fermigier (1986) remarks on the striking similarity between the narrator's estate in "The Horla" and Flaubert's mansion in Normandy. Jacques Bienvenu (1991) even suggested that the literary relation between Maupassant and Flaubert is in fact the allegorical point of focus of "The Horla." At a more formal level, Jameson's particular attention to the gridded description of the house located "between an alley way and a lane leading down to the river" in the fourth paragraph of *A Simple Heart* brings into focus the topographical consideration in the second paragraph of "The Horla" regarding the position of the diarist's house by the river.

whether or not the source of the disturbance is environmental or psychological. Eventually, the cluster of symptoms finds an etiology. The narrator manages to identify the origin of the disruption after reading an article describing an outbreak of collective psychosis in Brazil, in which he recognizes both his ailment ("The panicky inhabitants are leaving their homes, deserting their villages, abandoning their fields, claiming they are being pursued, possessed, controlled like cattle by invisible yet tangible beings" [Maupassant 2003, 189]) and a probable pathway ("Ah! I recall, I recall the glorious Brazilian three-master that sailed past my windows on May 8th" [Maupassant 2003, 190]), revealing in retrospect the fatidic nature of the picturesque procession of boats in the journal's first entry. What was initially in the background irrupts on the center stage to claim its share of reality and a name—the Horla.

Whatever the Horla is—a hallucination, a spiritual or elemental entity, or an environmental illness caused by a neurotoxin—its reality is unsettling, prophetic, and potentially world-ending, which prompts the diarist to declare the reign of man to be over. Notice here that the end does not come in the form of an extinction event. The terminal state *The Horla* envisions as its apocalypse is not the vision of a lawless world after history in which men behave like beasts. Rather, it has something to do with the loss of a dominion of humankind over the Earth. In the same way that humans have colonized the planet, a new species—the Horla—is about to colonize humanity: "man has killed the lion with an arrow, with a spear, with gunpowder; but the Horla will make man into what man has made the horse and of the ox: his chattel, his slave, and his food, by the sheer power of his will" (2003, 190. Modified translation). What is feared (and mourned) in this scenario is not so much the biological extinction of the human species than the loss of a universalist definition of the human promoted by the imperialist project. We are in a configuration where it is easier for the narrator to imagine the end of the human species than end of the colonialist project of mastery over other humans: the paradigm of humanity is either the kind of man the narrator is or would like to be, or it is game over.

Notice too how easily we go from the narrator's personal plight to the fate of humankind. What is at stake in the existential risk the Horla represents for the narrator is a very specific definition of the human as conqueror, master, and colonizer. It's not the end of the world, only the end of a narrative of mastery. In fact, nothing happens in the end and nothing gives the reader more assurance of the diarist's delusion.

The world can breathe easy. The Horla outbreak was just a bad psychotic episode. The pandemic threat, if there ever was one, was nothing but a scare. More importantly, the narrative of mastery whose collapse Maupassant briefly hallucinated remains unscathed. Civilizational collapse remains essentially speculative, without a definitive genre to hold on to: it could be a thought experiment just as well as it could be a bad dream. That said the story has indeed all the trappings of an outbreak narrative. It "begins with the identification of an emerging infection, includes discussion of the global networks throughout which it travels" (Wald 2008, 2) except that it doesn't end with a phase of containment. It is because the Horla has an unusual relation to writing.

On August 17, the narrator discovers that the disrupting presence reads: "I saw, yes, I saw with my own eyes another page rise and drop upon the preceding page as if moved by a finger. [...] I realized that *it* was there, it, sitting in my seat and reading" (2003, 189). This observation leads him to devise a baiting strategy, where he pretends to write and let the Horla read over his shoulder. In this moment of absorption and decoy, *we* are the Horla. We too read over the narrator's shoulder a pretend diary. We are the parasitical presence that entered the narrator's life and gained access to his inner thoughts, passing judgments on his written words, and that, in turn, the diarist delusion is in his relentless attempts to put an end to the dissymmetry between writing and reading. No matter what, the reader always outlives the writer, even if it is for the briefest moment.

The Horla outbreak also eludes containment efforts because of its relation to space. In virology, a chimera is "a new hybrid microorganism created by joining nucleic acid fragments from two or more different microorganisms in which each of at least two of the fragments contain essential genes necessary for replication" (Hill Jr. 2005). For Michel Serres (1994, 61–85), the Horla is a prepositional chimera: the impossible compound form of *hors* (out of, except, beside) and *là* (there). It is new to the world, less as an emerging entity that you can call infectious, than as an emerging property of a world where everything and everyone are unevenly connected. In "The Horla," connectivity is first a form and then a value. Its attributes can be both good and bad objects. Connectivity can create a sense of closeness, continuity, and prospects that integrates everything in the world as far as the eye can see into a mental landscape, as in the first entry of the diary: "Through my windows I can see the Seine [...] which runs from Rouen to Le Havre, crowded with passing boats"

(2003, 169). The connectivity that informs epidemiology on the other hand is bad news, or at least a source of news, fodder for a diary, for a *nouvelle* perhaps, that is, a short story. It is the kind of connectivity that you can't always see and that only becomes visible or legible after the fact as patterns, correlations, conjectures, and disruptions. It brings neither comfort nor intimacy.

By contrast with the first entry, whose sensorial vocabulary revolves predominantly around sight, on day 2 of his diary, the narrator intuits the existence of a world that is not primarily organized by vision and optical mastery: "Everything around us, everything we see without looking, everything we brush past without knowing it, everything we touch without feeling it, everything we encounter without distinguishing it— everything exerts rapid, surprising, and inexplicable effects on us, on our organs, and, through them, on our ideas and even on our hearts" (2003, 170). Here, touch is not understood as conveying relatability and nearness but vulnerability and contagion. It posits a world where totality is not the sum of voluntary actions born from intentions but the combination of two narrative logics: one that pertains to what germs "want"—usually expressed in the form of evolutionary microbiology and epidemiology—and the other that has to do with what humans want— traditionally captured by historiography and realist novels. Maupassant's narrator wants the (colonial) world he lives in without the (epidemiological) totality that comes with it—as if he had any choice in the matter.

If realism designates the belief held by narratives in the continuous existence of a world that is out there in the form of shared coordinates you can count on to tell the story of a nation, chide mavericks in need of a reality check, or conversely celebrate their visionary but ultimately self-destructive boldness (Hayot 2012, 124), then, epidemiological realism is not, in its first modality, about how realistic representations of epidemic events are. Rather, *it is about a sense of narrative continuity in a world governed by epidemiological principles that apply everywhere and explain everything that falls within their purview* (Fig. 2.1).

Some versions of epidemiological realism, like the One Health model with its integrative, equitable, ecocentric, transdisciplinary, multi-scalar and planetary approach and the heavy visual investment of its promotional material in orbs and other spherical shapes, are world building. Other versions, like the one intuited by Montaigne in his writing about the fate of the indigenous population of the Americas in the wake of the

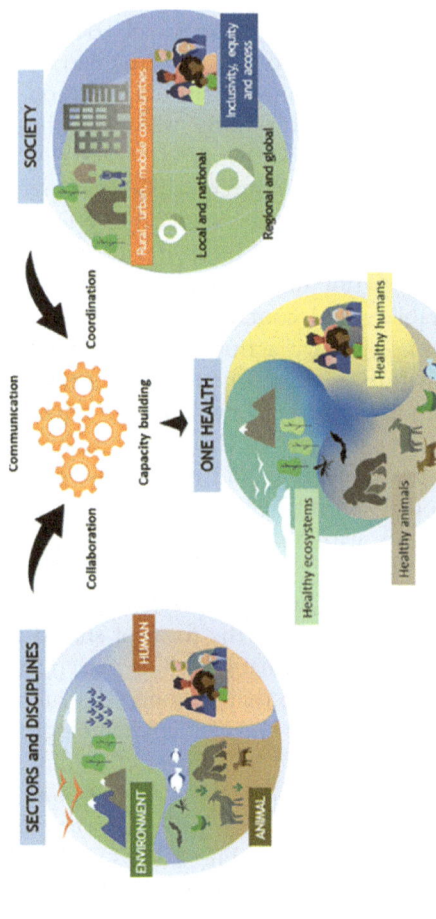

Fig. 2.1 "One Health" paradigm visual investment in orbs and other spherical shapes (One Health High-Level Expert Panel 2022)

Columbian exchange five hundred years ago, are world negating: "Our world has just discovered another [...] no less great, full, and well-limbed than itself, yet so new and so infantile that it is still being taught its A B C; [...] I am much afraid that we shall have greatly hastened the decline and ruin of this new world by our contagion" (Montaigne 1958, 908–909. See also Crosby 1972). To be fair, the meaning of the word "contagion" in these lines is not epidemiological. It merely designates a negative form of contact in early modern French. Nevertheless, the epidemiological afterlives of the term use by Montaigne in one of his most important essays on the New World can be interpreted as soft evidence that the realist affirmation of a worldview that encompasses everything on the planet cannot be separated from European logics of territorial expansion.

A diagnostic footnote in André Fermigier's edition (1986, 75) attempts to settle what's unsettling about Maupassant's story: "Maupassant has already reported that type of negative hallucination in *Letter of a Madman* (1885). One could imagine that he suffered from them himself." The Horla is in the diarist's head just like it was in the authors' sick mind. It is a symptom of an underlying venereal condition left untreated and manifesting itself in the form of cognitive impairment in an otherwise masterful narrative. Case closed. The last sentence of the diary indicates that the narrator has resolved to take his own life after realizing that he can neither escape nor contain the global scourge. In the first version of "The Horla" (1886), the narrator turned himself in and shared his story with an alienist. The trusted doctor closes the narrative loop for the reader by orchestrating the dissemination of the strange story among colleagues in a clinical salon of sorts but at the end seems reluctant to close the case altogether. In this version, the outbreak is more or less contained by narrative conventions as fiction.

What distinguishes fiction from ordinary experience, Jacques Rancière explains (2017, 7), is not a lack of reality but a supplement of rationality. There is more in the stories we tell and read than there is to reality, because even at its most descriptive, fiction offers a rationale for how things are, how they fall into place or through the cracks, follow pattern or go off on a tangent. In that sense, epidemiology is but a version of the fictional rationale that operates on the heuristic premise that, in the words of virologist Philip Mortimer, "an outbreak like a story should have a coherent plot. In classical drama. Aristotle required there be unity of time, place and action" (2003, 448). Or in those of historian of medicine, Charles Rosenberg writing at the height of the AIDS crisis in the US: "Epidemics […] follow a plot line of increasing and revelatory tension, move to a crisis of individual and collective character, then drift toward closure" (1989, 2). It also means that if non- or pre-epidemiological sources and interpretive methodologies have something relevant to say about the epidemiological present, it is not at the level of what they get intuitively right about emerging relations, or the exemplarity of a case. Rather it is to the extent that what epidemiology is, does, and is believed to be capable of has been modeled after a story-telling tradition, and that this mode of accounting for the world too is an object of ongoing contestation—or Samuel Weber's preferred terms, friction (2022).[2]

In practice, however, epidemiological realities too can lack in narrative coherence. The foot-and-mouth disease outbreak on English farms in 2001, Annemarie Mol and John Law (2011) argue, was not in the symptomatic lesions present on the foot and mouth of the cattle; it was not in the labs running the tests for the disease; it was not assignable to the actual spread or risk of spread from a farm to the other either. If the disease was anywhere, it was in an absence of shared coordinates. Non-identity does not leave us with a problem of representation, vision, or perspective on the world, but with a problem of coordination between practices: the clinic deals with bodies, the lab deals with specimens, and epidemiology deals with records. Clinicians identify symptoms, lab workers isolate microscopic entities in samples, and epidemiologists reconstitute likely pathways of infections. It is this absence of shared coordinates that Maupassant's outbreak narrative intuits in the madness of his narrator and restitutes as non-fiction by way of a faux diary defying the rationales that its commitment to evidentiary thinking solicits nevertheless. This is the second modality of epidemiological realism: *epidemiological events are not immediately available to us as objects of inquiry and concern but only through the lens of narrative and visual conventions that either substantiate or deflate claims to crisis.*

Nestled within the narrative principles Rosenberg and Mortimer assigned to epidemic events, *the third modality of epidemiological realism* exemplified by "The Horla" *corresponds to the operational frame within*

---

[2] Frictions, or frictional narratives—by contradistinction with fictions and fictional narratives—"incorporate elements that designate existing entities, persons, things, and places, but transpose them into a realm where their significance can be altered and developed without being crushed by the weight of reality" (Weber 2022, 90).

which security experts anticipating on the next pandemic crisis and its impact on political institutions and social infrastructures learn from scenario-based exercises. With great storytelling power comes important responsibilities. Professor Dame Sally Davies, UK Special Envoy on Antimicrobial Resistance, began the talk she delivered in January 2021 at the Emory School of Medicine with a confession: "I never tell politicians what to do. I ask myself: What story will they buy into? Which fact will they listen to?" She presents herself as a modern-day Scheherazade, whose expert narrative skills are put to good use to postpone public health disasters and defuse epidemiological timebombs. In the biopreparedness context, fiction doesn't lack reality. It beckons future events waiting to happen in an ecology of threats. To paraphrase Catherine Belling, this modality of epidemiological realism eventuates in stories that are not primarily intended to serve as a testimonial record. Instead they "remind us [...] of something we cannot remember in order to prepare us for a future we cannot adequately predict" (2009, 71).

With its hint at a dark version of present-day globalization, where exotic viruses are just a commercial flight away, "The Horla" prefigures what Elizabeth Povinelli wittily calls "ghoul health" (2006, 77–83). Ghoul health is the thing that global health nightmares are made of. But it also is the kind of nightmares the global North likes to have—because it is easier to envision exotic superbugs bringing down an entire system in the most spectacular (and hemorrhagic) manners than the cruddy accumulation of entrenched health disparities that very system is built on. And because in the end it is less politically embarrassing to blame an epidemic crisis on an invisible entity than on an inadequate supply of ventilators or Personal Protective Equipment.

The Horla's prophecy anticipates on the time in which we will live under constant threat, surrounding ourselves with projection models even though nothing happens. And when something finally does, it will still catch us off guard, unprepared, flailing for genre (Berlant 2018), unable to adjust. As such, *the fourth modality of epidemiological realism lends expression to forms of hyperawareness that at time can be difficult to bear.* In "The Horla," this expressivity ranges from the humble compulsion to record everything noteworthy in a diary, to more ambitious lyrical moments ("how about the butterfly? A flying blossom! I picture one the size of a hundred universes, with wings whose shape, beauty, color, and motion I cannot express" [2003, 192]). This modality is essentially affective and genre-bending. As such, it is positioned on the receptive end of temporal relations in search of a plotline. It registers and assesses disturbances in the conventions of relating random misfortunes to systemic affliction, and vice versa.

Maybe the Horla is less an imagined threat than a response to the threat. What if the narrator was the threat to the home and the Horla the purifying plague that drives the intruder out before he contaminates the household? What if it was precisely the kind of pestilence that puts an end to someone's claims to kinship? The narrator has ancestral claims to the familial estate. He has roots attaching him "to the soil where his forebears were born and died" but bears no fruits. Because of his intruding celibacy in an otherwise reproductive setting, he doesn't really belong in the place he still calls home. In which case "The horla" reads like the story of someone who has internalized a form of undesirability.

Or maybe "The Horla" is the fable of an estate owner who became allergic to his own lifestyle, the nineteenth-century equivalent of Carol White's undiagnosed reaction to her suburbanite milieu in Todd Haynes's film *Safe* (1995).[3] At any rate, like the environmental toxicity that finds a notional expression in the contested category of sick building syndrome or Multiple chemical sensitivity (MCS), the Horla "cannot be adequately understood by answering the question, 'Is it real or not?'" (Murphy 2006, 18). The Horla outbreak may not be real in the sense that it is at once a figment of the narrator's psychotic imagination and a byproduct of his storytelling abilities but it has tragic consequences on others. In a desperate attempt to both contain and destroy the Horla, the narrator ends up destroying his mansion by fire, killing his staff in the process.

Real or not, the Horla leaves reality "in the thrall of a specter" (Caduff 2015, 3). It is already at home in what Rosenberg considered to be an era of abusive language, where "every day we hear of 'epidemics' of alcoholism, drug addiction, and automobile accidents." He adds rather dismissively: "The intent is clear enough: to clothe certain undesirable yet blandly tolerated social phenomena in the emotional urgency associated with a 'real' epidemic" (1989, 1). Thirty years later, the purism of the distinction Rosenberg wished to maintain between real epidemics and rhetorical epidemics seems almost inappropriate. Any negative relation can

---

[3] It's not the first time *Safe* has elicited a comparison with nineteenth-century French literature. For Roddey Reid (1998), Carol White is a twentieth-century version of Emma Bovary, "the original 'hysterical' housewife driven to suicide" by her bourgeois lifestyle.

become an object of epidemiological knowledge: communicable and non-communicable diseases, addiction, toxicity, domestic violence, heat stress, depression, eating disorder, wildfire, dementia… etc. At its most abstract, epidemiology is a science of negative relationality that finds a concrete expression as death, injury, and morbidity, but also more elusively as increased risk, loss of income, and reduced economic productivity. In that sense, epidemiological realism is about the challenge of representing negative relations and living with them—or, of representing negative relations in order to live with them. Epidemiological realism asks us to commit cognitive resources to thinking about what it means to live with negative relations.

CHAPTER 3

Facing Toxicity (New York City Health Department 2019; Health Canada 2010; FDA 2018)

Abstract With its focus on environmental toxicity, this vignette is an illustration of what epidemiology can do for us. It tracks down the source of poisoning but it is also what redirects our eyes toward relations that a certain version of realism had relegated to the background. In turn, and because it draws attention to the invisibility of backdrops against which stories ought to take place, more or less independently, epidemiology returns us to the images we entrust the story of our lives to.

Keywords Body horror · BPA · Environmental toxicity · Lead poisoning · Photorealism · Tobacco · Vaping · Viscerality

By now, BPA, or bisphenol A, has become a familiar presence—a household name dare I say. It is high on the list of invisible entities that denizens of post-industrial societies have learned to spot around them, hiding in plain sight in the comfort of their well-appointed home and the transparency of the most mundane objects—not unlike the Horla in Maupassant short story. BPA is an organic compound used, for instance, to produce solid transparent plastic. Molecular bioscientist Patricia Hunt identified its endocrine disrupting properties in the late 1990s, when a control group of mice started to present a high rate of chromosomal abnormalities in their egg cells that could only be explained by the plastic environment in which the control group was conditioned (Landecker 2015). The disturbance was registered within the experimental setting at the level of the distinction between background and foreground, that is, between what is inert and what is active. It revealed the neutral space of the lab—a space within which objectivity depends on standard protocols of isolation—to have its own environmental dimension as a milieu of life. But it also revealed that the plastic consuming control group outside the lab setting as yet another test group enrolled in an open-ended experiment where untested chemicals make up the stuff of everyday life.

The BPA vignette is an illustration of what epidemiology can do for us. It tracks down the source of poisoning but it is also what redirects our eyes toward relations that a certain version of realism had relegated to the background. In turn, and because it draws attention to the invisibility of backdrops against which stories ought to take place, more or less independently, epidemiology returns us to the images we entrust the story of our lives to. The lead poisoning awareness campaign created by the New York City Health department in 2019 asks us to believe that the world is a toxic place ("Lead in peeling paint poisons children") but that it could be a safer one ("Tell your landlord to fix peeling paint," "Wash floors, windowsills, hands, and toys often"). Its epidemiological realism is not what purifies our representations of the world in an effort to transmit information and reabsorb the background noise. It is what binds toxicity to the representation of human events (Fig. 3.1).

In this particular image, lead toxicity is less a chemical relation between bodies and objects, than a visual relation between the inquisitive toddler chewing on a bright toy while soliciting the camera, and the immaculate white background that insures the legibility of the poster's message. The red and black letters that make up that message are not the only eye-catching marks on the wall. Another inscription enjoys the same level of visual definition and legibility in the form of a flaking in the paint that recalls the conventional transparency of the background to its materiality as a milieu. The crisp lines of the dent in the wall behind the toddler are simultaneously descriptive and narrative. They gesture toward the patterns of toxic incidence that the campaign seeks to interrupt. As a sign of wear and tear, the flaking also adds temporal depth to the instantaneous image (a photographic second in the life of a toddler). There may be no toxic event to speak of per se, when it comes to lead toxicity. The dented image, however, speaks to the duration that allows poisonings to occur.

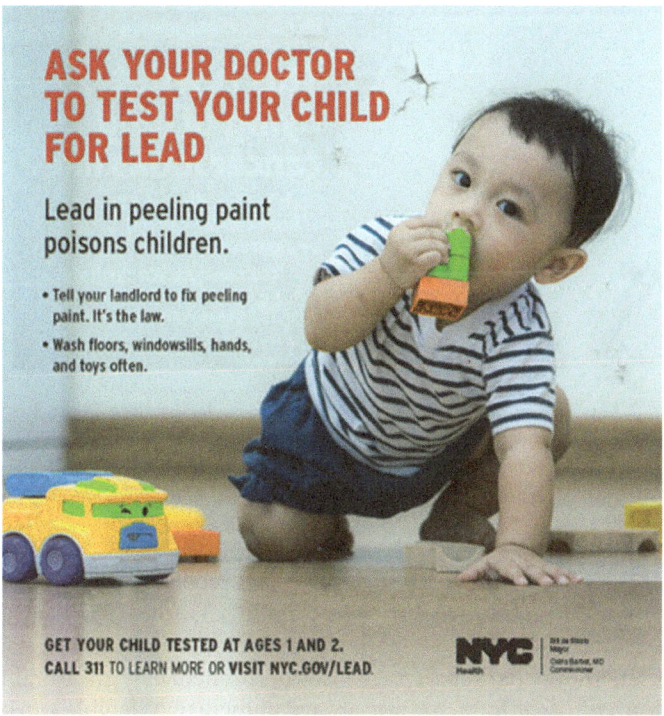

Fig. 3.1 New York City Health. "Ask your doctor to test your child for lead"

In a different visual register, the images affixed to tobacco products in Europe and Canada are not just images of "what dying of cancer looks like." They intend to reveal the true nature of what's in the box. They are statement about the proven link between tobacco product and carcinogenic effects, or between tobacco cytotoxicity and the bodies that bear this chemical burden. The emaciated and hairless likeness of Barb Tarbox (1961–2003) on Canadian cigarettes packaging is what toxicity looks like too. The portrait on a box is a distant medial memory of the funerary origins of the genre in Roman Egypt. But here, it is also a statement about the toxicity of the box content. The image on the box itself becomes a box in its attempt to close in the temporal gap between exposure to carcinogenic substances and the clinical manifestation of cytotoxicity in the form of a cancer diagnosis. The link between image and toxicity on the box of

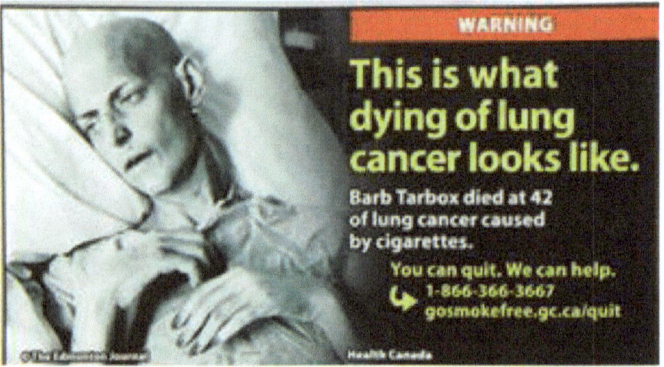

Fig. 3.2 "This is what dying of lung cancer looks like." Barb Tarbox photographed by Greg Southam. Health Labels for Cigarettes and Little Cigars, Health Canada 2010. Material republished with the express permission of Edmonton Journal, a division of Postmedia Network Inc.

cigarettes is sanctioned by epidemiologists and recognized by tort law but it is not the case for all toxic relations (Jain 2013, 190–191) (Fig. 3.2).

Toxicity—and this goes for tobacco toxicity—is aniconic. It does not look like anything. Its impact is not always immediately measurable in a population and its effects are not always immediately legible on bodies. Its relation to visuality is a matter of conventions of relating invisibility to visibility. What's invisible in images of what tobacco toxicity looks like is the inside of the body. It is invisible because it is inside. What's invisible in images of what e-cigarette or vaping product toxicity looks like is the invisibility of what the European Respiratory Society described as unknown but not safe either (Hamberger and Halpern-Felsher 2020, 379) (Fig. 3.3).

In 2018, the U.S. Surgeon General and the Food and Drug Administration (FDA) commissioner declared the use of e-cigarettes among adolescent an epidemic. That same year, the FDA developed a campaign around a series of digitally altered portraits. The digital alterations are minimal and yet arresting. They introduce what appears to be patterns of scar tissue on young faces, especially around the mouth and nose area. The skin lesions are not understood to be real in a clinical sense. They anticipate on the emergence of adverse relations between adolescent bodies and long-term effects of ECIG use before the future shows up in

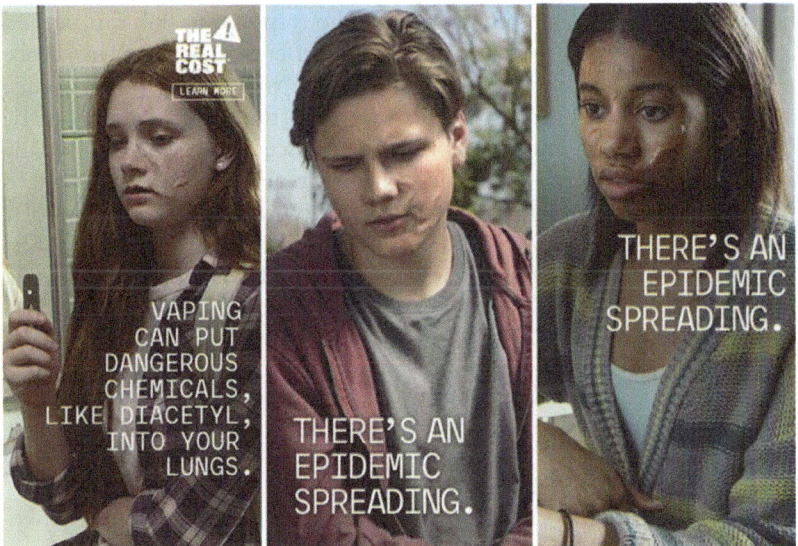

Fig. 3.3 "The Real Cost" Campaign. HHS.gov

the form of another public health disaster.[1] Their photorealism also anticipates on the state of affairs in which chemicals and bodies will be linked
by the images of damaged organs and body parts used in traditional anti-
tobacco products campaigns. In the meantime, the gap between indexical
and digital image will have to be filled by visual tropes borrowed from
the playbook of body horror cinema. By tapping into the visual repertoire of unwanted bodily transformations, the digitally altered portraits of
"The Real Cost" Campaign visualize uncertainty by "visceralizing" risk—
at the risk, some may object, of undermining the entire cautionary effort
of classic anti-tobacco imagery built on the truth-value of pulmonary
nodules, decaying teeth, and ulcerated lips. But so far, no objections have
been raised.

Visceralization is a source of visual discomfort that both internalizes
and exposes. It is a way to internalize the difference between the unknown
and the unsafe, between probability and cases, and between incidence

---

[1] In 2019, the CDC reported 2500 cases of acute respiratory failure related to e-
cigarette or vaping product use (Hamberger and Halpern-Felsher 2020).

and event, now and then, if and when. The response to risk can be said to be visceral precisely because the elusive difference between incidence and event is lived with in the meantime, while waiting for the difference to resorb itself at some point, even if at time the thought of it can be too much to take in and keep inside. The visceral anecdote quoted by Michel Leiris (1930, 261) in a meditative piece on the art of early modern anatomical illustration comes to mind: "A woman caught a glimpse of a disembowelled ox in the process of being gutted at a butcher stand. She experienced such disgust that she almost fainted. When pressed to talk about the fit that came over her, she asked 'Are our bodies filled with that much vileness too?' The answer she received persuaded her to let herself starve to death."

CHAPTER 4

Facing Exemplarity (*Still Alice* 2014)

Abstract Alice's story, in the film adaptation of Lisa Genoa's 2007 novel *Still Alice* (2014), might be exemplary but it is not necessarily epidemiologically representative. Early onset Alzheimer disease (AD) represents less than 0.5% of diagnosed cases. With its clear genetic markers, Alice's Alzheimer lends its exemplarity to the localization argument in the epidemiology of AD and yet her imaginary fate is also a study in entangled relations between narrative and visual forms.

Keywords Alzheimer disease · Biography · Medical imaging · Portraiture · *Still Alice* (film), suicide ideation · Utermohlen, William

The realism of Sabrina Raaf's installation "Breath Cultures" (1999) consists in a colorful display of bacterial and fungal growths set in petri dishes layered with nutrient gel. Each microbial recording captured and developed the oral flora contained in the breath of a group of participants from all over the world, each matched with a voice recording from the same participants answering the same narrative prompt: to share in their own language childhood memories of their favorite candy (a food group known to significantly alter the oral flora) (Raaf 2006). Another way to frame this experiment is to say with Bratton, that "Breath Cultures" invites sitters to see themselves and presents themselves to the world less as "an interiority occupied by private voice and experience and more a medium through which the physical world signifies itself" (2021, 35–36). The realism of Raaf's installation is epidemiological insofar as it is invested in matching breaths, voices, idioms, and the stories that live somewhere in or in-between them. Its "object-scene," to go back to Berlant (2011, 52), is perhaps less the candy itself than the dual meaning of the word "culture" in laboratory science and social science, and with it, the prospect of capturing the infinite distance that exists between biology and biography in the form of a microbiological portrait of sorts.

All it takes for a sonogram to become a portrait and, in turn, alter what counts as portraiture, is a frame and a wall. In a pinch, a fridge magnet will do. In early modern European painting, frames on walls are the object of intense formal experiments. They set images apart. They also draw lines in space that can be crossed under special circumstances and impinged upon by protruding objects to create dazzling visual conundrums. Art historian Victor Stoichita explains that "the closest an image reaches to the real space by impinging upon it, the more its supra-temporal nature is called into question: it becomes a 'fallen' image as soon as it relinquishes the beyond, that is, the realm of an imaginary eternity, in order to invade the down here, the world of mortals" (1997, 62). But even as a fallen image, a framed sonogram signals that we have come to accept its visual terms and with them the claims of medical imaging on our lives insofar as lives are framed and reframed by biomedicine, public health, biostatistics; or insofar as lives have a lifespan and a life-expectancy, and insofar as they can be lost to diagnoses and prognoses before being lost to death.

In the opening scene of the film adaptation of Lisa Genoa's 2007 novel, *Still Alice* (Richard Glatzer and Wash Westmoreland 2014), Alice's birthday situates an impending diagnosis in a lifespan. It is a marker of time, an occasion for celebration, a gathering, a future memory in the making; all things that early onset Alzheimer disease (AD) will both reframe and disrupt. Alice's life has become the place where AD appears legible as a series of symptoms embedded in her cognitive unravelling. Alice's diagnosis is established and confirmed through a series of clinical tests: a verbal cognitive impairment assessment followed by a genetic panel of blood tests and a PET scan of her brain revealing amyloid buildup consistent with Alzheimer disease.

In a review of the film, a clinician voiced concerns regarding the somewhat unrealistic expectations set by the portrayal of Alice's diagnosis, noting that "Amyloid PET scans are a relatively new test and are very helpful in the diagnosis of dementia. However, they are not approved by any insurance plan, including Medicare, and they cost over $5,000 out-of-pocket. Currently [in 2015] they are done mostly at research centers for those who are willing to pay for them, but that is very infrequent" (Devere 2015, 44). The reservations are duly noted but my interest in the scene lies somewhere else; chiefly, in the fact that medical images shed their diagnostic identity all the time. They seemingly escape manila envelopes, folding cabinets and document shredders to find their ways in plotlines as yet another biographical moving part to contend with, when it comes to negotiating expectations, unpredictability, the unknown, and the invisible.

The amyloid PET scan is part of a narrative sequence of shots and counter-shots that suggests that the high-tech rendition of Alice's damaged brain also functions as a portrait—if indeed a portrait is the image that stands for someone in their absence, signaling that the sense of immediacy that is to be borne by the body is not currently available. It is not necessarily an image of the face, as in the medieval and early modern escutcheons tradition (Belting 2014). Or from a different angle, one could say that the diagnostic image functions like a portrait because it introduces a new container in the series that locates modern interiority in "the subject's presence to itself as a spatial enclosure, room, tomb, or crypt in which the voice echoes as in a cave" (De Man 1984, 288). If the echoing voice in *Still Alice* is neurological, then the amyloid buildup in the brain is her, if not hers, or at least a version of herself. It is only a matter of time before what has been deciphered on the inside by clinical tests as a physiological and genetic marker consistent with an AD diagnosis finds a clinical expression on the "outside" and eventually takes over (Fig. 4.1).

The biographical delay between the presence of physiological and genetic markers and the absence of clinical symptoms of dementia they forecast is materialized by the series of self-portraits painted by William Utermohlen in the wake of his AD diagnosis in 1995. According to a clinical study of his artworks published in *The Lancet*, symptoms of cognitive impairment are detectable in Utermohlen's late production but not to the point of precluding the very existence of these paintings. The authors observe that "a portrait, painted at 65 years, is more abstract in nature and reflects the fact that the realism of his previous work is no longer attainable. [...] This dramatic shift in style and approach is consistent with the

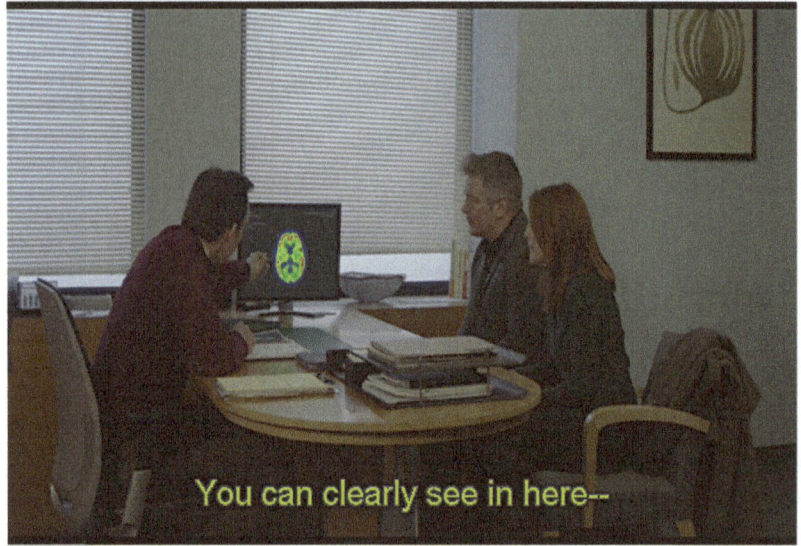

You can clearly see in here--

Fig. 4.1   Alice confronting her amyloid PET scan. *Still Alice*

production of other abstract paintings the following year. Here, perspective and depth are lost but form and colour are still used in a creative and original manner" (Crutch et al. 2001, 2130–2131). The clinical legibility of Utermohlen's artistic trajectory is the result of a montage juxtaposing different type of visuals—a diagram, a magnetic resonance coronal image, and artworks—and positing a negative convergence between them. Something symptomatic can be detected in the artist's turn toward abstraction, not as the result of an intentional engagement with a form of aesthetic expression and the history of painting, but as an unmistakable sign of decline in his ability to process spatial relations. It means that a point will come in the progression of the symptoms where Utermohlen's artwork won't be realist enough to respond to the clinical signs of the progression of the disease. Regardless, the biographical delay is not explained away by the portraits but fleshed out by them.

Because of their very existence, because they were painted and painted with noticeable differences in their execution, rather than not painted at all, Utermohlen's late self-portraits are placeholders for the AD etiological conundrum. "Localization theorists," Margaret Lock explains, "visualize

AD as a demonstrable neuropathological entity whereas entanglement theorists are more inclined to understand AD as an emergent process—the product of contextualized individual biologies and life experiences culminating in the clinical expression of the phenomenon of AD/dementia" (2013, 13). On the one hand, the case of Utermohlen's self-portraits as proxy-picture of his cognitive decline speaks to the localization hypothesis. On the other, the painter's aesthetic trajectory toward abstraction offers a different version of the entanglement hypothesis that extends to broad categories in art history and the history of painting as medium of self-expression.

If *Still Alice* treats the diagnostic image (the Amyloid PET scans) as a portrait, one could say that *The Lancet* study treats Utermohlen's self-portraits as a form of diagnostic imaging. Utermohlen's self-portraits and Alice's fictional biography are places where knowledge about AD is produced. However, what is perhaps the most striking narrative feature of Alice's life is that the autobiographical scenario—one could also speak of an autobiographical ideation—is a direct threat to her life. Coming to terms with the diagnosis and its impact on her family and her career, but also registering the extent of the degenerative potential that the diagnosis brings, Alice sets up a time bomb in the form of video recorded message from herself to her "then-self" (Post 1995). The detonator consists in a series of questions probing narrative standards of continuity and consistency—What is the name of your oldest daughter? What street do you live on? What month is your birthday?—with the implication that stories that stray too much from these biographical standards are not to be told and thus not to be lived. And so, the recorded message stipulates, should you fail to rehearse the basic plot of your life, go the drawer, take all the pills, and don't tell anybody. It's time to end the story (Fig. 4.2).

The time bomb set by now-Alice works on the assumption that time will erase her mastery over language. Then-Alice can't understand what is implied by the directives, only follow them. Indeed, the video recording tucked away in the computer memory does not come with a pedagogy of reading attached to it. The autobiographical ticking device, however, is not foolproof. It fizzles when then-Alice fails to follow her own advanced directives, at which point AD takes over. Then-Alice's failure to follow through is not a competent reversal of the previous decision. It defuses the sense that something even happened along with the assurance of what an event is supposed to look like, whether it is shaped by cognitive glitches, projects, deadlines, and milestones. And yet, the glitch in

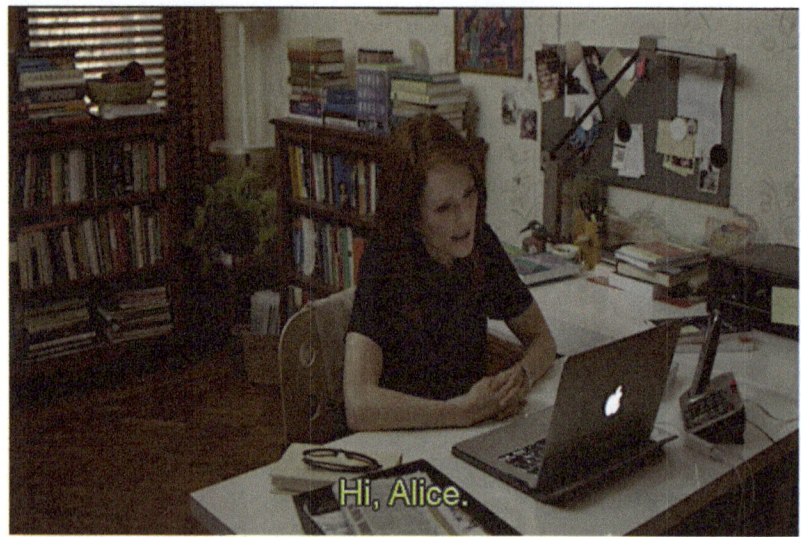

Fig. 4.2 Now-Alice recording a message to then-Alice

the suicide narrative buys Alice more biographical time to be lived in uncharted narrative spaces. The unconsented plot twist seeks a different solution to cognitive decline by alleviating some of the pressure put on the notion of narrative agency from the biographical equation that is Alice, now and then.

Legal documents aim at interpreting and modifying the social relations they represent, by convention; by convention, fictions do not, but conventional borders and preset filters remain porous. Bioethicists read fiction and engage with it by narrating cases and putting forward arguments. In turn, fiction produced across generic and disciplinary boundaries reabsorbs societal aspirations that biomedical futures are expected to meet (Squier 2004). In bioethics, fiction is characterized by its absorption properties. The use of fictional material as a testing ground and as a source of cautionary tales does not require an IRB. And yet, stories we tell about dementia can be dangerous and do harm too, for instance, when they fail to imagine "what counts as evidence that living is taking place" in the absence of narrative agency (Berlant and Prosser 2011, 185–186. See also

Chambers 2017, 173–174). *Still Alice* holds on to a project of person-hood against the threat of erasure, while it simultaneously challenges assumptions regarding narratives of personhood.

In this version of a non-self-destructive ending, AD represents the new frontier of biography and memoir writing. It represents the limit against which to imagine what living a life would look like in the absence of narrative agency. *Still Alice* allows us to envision AD in its ramification beyond the moment of the initial clinical encounter in a relational perspective. Alice's memory loss received an unambiguous medical diagnosis but what AD means to her takes time to sink in—the duration of the movie—and will be recovered in a language of loss, regrets, and closure. What it means to have AD is always already embedded in personal and professional expectations scripting the life course and in assumptions regarding what it is to be someone and to no longer be that person.

Alice's story might be exemplary in that respect, but it is not epidemiologically representative. Early onset Alzheimer represents less than 0.5% of diagnosed cases. With its clear genetic markers, Alice's Alzheimer lends its exemplarity to the localization argument (that seeks to visualize AD "as a demonstrable neuropathological entity"), and yet her imaginary fate is also a study in entangled relations between narrative and visual forms.

It is hard to imagine how *Still Alice* could have ever been an autobiographical account, at least up to a certain point. By the end of a story that could never have been hers entirely, Alice is no longer Alice Howland, a white woman in her early fifties, a wife, a mother, and a distinguished college professor at an elite institution. Even though she is still alive at the end, Alice has already lost a version of her life to an early onset Alzheimer disease (AD) diagnosis, because of the loss of narrative and cognitive agency that characterize the progression of the disease. Here, the chiasm is not between biology and biography, even though etiological hypotheses linking AD to infections and inflammations exist, but between what it means to have a life and what it means to lose it to a rare form of inherited neurodegenerative disease.

CHAPTER 5

Picturing Incidence (Clara Jacobi 1689; Stromae 2015)

Abstract Faces of real men and women standing for the difficult conversations they had to have are the main visual trope of a 2010 French campaign, encouraging friends, family members, and coworkers to talk about breast cancer screening. There is nothing particularly remarkable about that structure of address unless one remembers that fifty years earlier, the public image of cancer in posters endorsed by the French Ministry of Health consisted mostly of allegorical formulas: a four-headed hydra slayed by a floating sword, a giant crab crushed by a disembodied fist or a spear that came from nowhere, and stylized silhouettes of warriors waging an invisible war. Vignette 5 investigates what it means and what it takes to put a face on cancer in the epidemiological present.

Keywords Cancer · Cancer culture · Jacobi, Clara · Portraiture · Self-awareness · Stromae

Faces of real men and women standing for the difficult conversations they had to have are the main visual trope of a 2010 French campaign, encouraging friends, family members, and coworkers to talk about breast cancer screening. There is nothing particularly remarkable about that structure of address unless one remembers that fifty years earlier, the public image

V. Bruyere, *Epidemiological Realism*, Palgrave Studies in Literature, Science and Medicine,
https://doi.org/10.1007/978-3-031-68517-0_5

of cancer in posters endorsed by the French Ministry of Health consisted mostly of allegorical formulas: a four-headed hydra slayed by a floating sword, a giant crab crushed by a firm fist or an ancient spear that came from nowhere, or stylized silhouettes of warriors waging an invisible war. There is no room for vulnerability in these images suggesting root force and strength. There is no acknowledgment of suffering either. It is as if cancer did not even take place in a life or a lifetime, had a duration made of remissions and relapses. Its existence in the verbal and visual lexicon of public health seems to be primarily a trigger in response to which a war is being waged (Figs. 5.1 and 5.2).

A cursory search for early modern images of cancer in the U.S. National Library of Medicine (NLM) digital collection reveals that putting a face on cancer or the conversation about cancer is not an entirely new rhetorical gesture. Among the few documents retrieved is an unattributed seventeenth-century Dutch engraving of a surgical patient, Clara Jacobi. Clara is seen in profile, first with a melon-size tumor protruding from her neck, and a second time without the tumor. In this image, cancer has the visual reality of a foreign body. It exists in a sequence within a surgical imaginary of extraction as a conspicuous mass to be removed. The mass itself might not have been cancerous by today's oncological standards, perhaps it is an enlarged cyst but it is obviously too late for a biopsy to be conducted. Instead of a retrospective diagnosis, the engraving and its bibliometric tagging with the word "cancer" invite us to reconstitute another story: even as Clara's excised tumor sits between two versions of herself, with and without cancer, her likeness survived on the edge of anonymity as the indelible trace of her encounter with cancer. Clara's cancer is conspicuous. It is part of her but it is not clear whether or not there is room for her to "have cancer" or "face cancer." Her portrait is incidental. We have an image of her face because cancer happens to be on her face. Another way to put it would be to say that first there is cancer, then there is Clara. If there is such a thing as Clara's cancer, it occupies a biographical space that doesn't exist (Fig. 5.3).

Cancer in cancer portraiture names an oncological reality but also the encounter—and sometimes non-encounter—between the image and the body. This is true of the portraits painted between 1836 and 1852 by Cantonese artist Lam Qua at the request of American physician Peter Parker. Just like for Clara, the monstrous presence of the tumors on the face of Qua's sitters warrants their anonymous encounter with a form of representation to which they would not have had access otherwise. In a

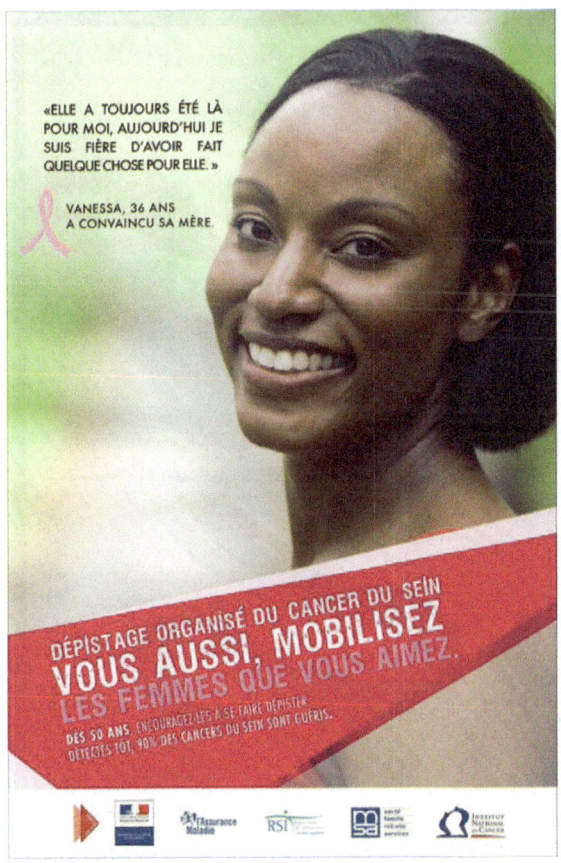

Fig. 5.1 Top right-hand corner: "She has always been there for me, today I am proud to have done something for her." "Vanessa, 36 years old, convinced her mother." Bottom script: "Organized Breast Cancer Screening. You too, mobilize the women you love. As early as age 50, encourage them to be screened. When detected early, 90% of breast cancers are cured." October 2010 breast cancer awareness campaign by Cespharm (educational branch of the French National Pharmacy Association) and the French National Cancer institute (INCa) (Photography: Daniel H. Bailey. Courtesy of the Institut national du cancer [Campagne de dépistage des cancers du sein de 2010])

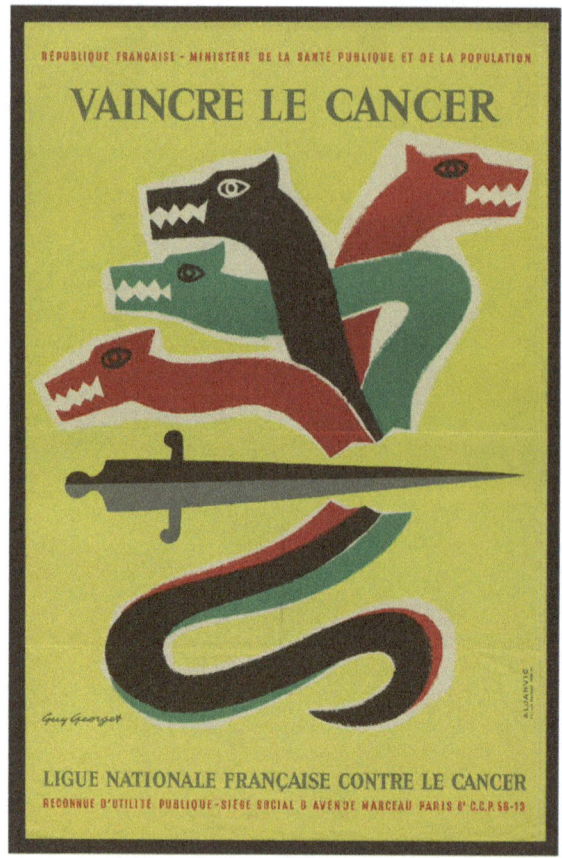

Fig. 5.2 "Defeating Cancer." French Republic, Ministry of Public Health and of the Population. French National League against Cancer. Lithograph after G. Georget, printed in colors. 1960. 59.9 × 39.5 cm

paradoxical twist on the conventions of portraiture, the tumor portraits do show someone's face, someone who assumes the countenance of a portrait sitting but only to portray a pivotal moment: "the moment at which [...] physical bodies are about to stop looking like the portraits that captured them" (Hayot 2009, 110). Clara's portrait too memorializes the surgeon's gesture. The engraving isolates the tumor leaving no signs of the patient's awareness regarding what has been done to her. As in Lam

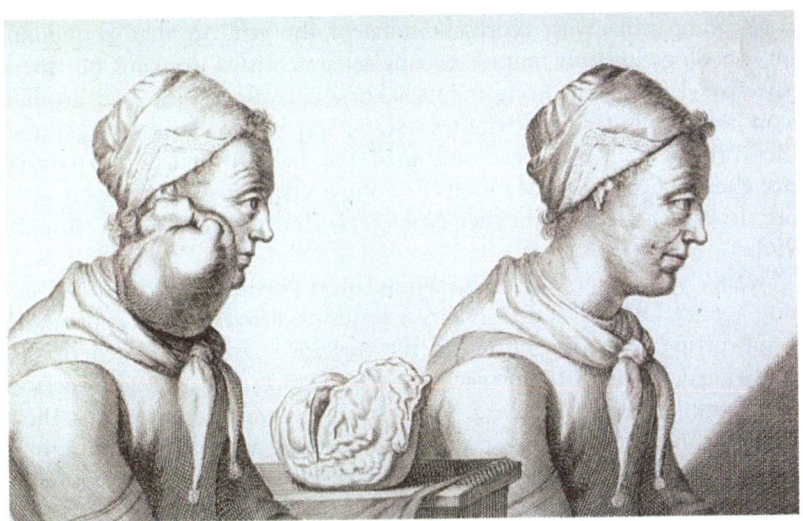

Fig. 5.3   Clara Jacobi. Netherlands, 1689. Engraving. 28 × 25 cm. National Library of Medicine

Qua tumor portraits, there is no legible signs regarding her subjective awareness of the tumor or of its absence. Portraiture here is not the visual repository of a sense of self awareness. Or to put it differently, subjective awareness is not the locus of a relation between face, cancer, and patient. Incidence is. Clara's surgery barely left any visible mark on her likeness, save for part of a missing earlobe and, of course, for the existence of the engraving itself. There is no scar to be located in Lam Qua's portraits either, for the obvious reason that they are portrait painted before the surgical interventions. Unless the erasure of the tumor-free patients, who can only exist in the register of portraiture through cancer, is understood as a pictorial form of scarred tissue.

Clara's portrait makes claim to a form of immediacy and self-recognition she probably did not even know she was entitled to, because there was no platform available for her to "have cancer," or "face up to it." Three centuries later, the survival of her diffracted portrait acts as a reminder that, in the same way that not all cancers are visible and solid, clinical representations of cancer as a cellular pathology are not always compatible with representations of the self. In that configuration, oncology and portraiture occupy separate visual domains but their respective claims to the body and its likeness nevertheless intersect around secondary public-facing attributes—scars, scarfs, hairlessness, wigs, and other prosthetics—that have redefined the field of cancer portraiture since the publication of Matuschka's controversial post-mastectomy self-portrait on the cover of the *New York Time Magazine* in August 1993.

Twenty years later, the Mimi Foundation partnered with the advertising agency Leo Burnett to realize a series of diffracted cancer portraits by subverting the conventions of the makeover scenario. Each of the twenty participants in the project was transformed and over-accessorized while keeping their eyes closed. Each was photographed twice, first their eyes shut, unaware of what was done to their face, and then a second time as they discover the unexpected transformation. Each shot is dated and timed to the second—hence the title: *If Only for a Second / Ne serait-ce qu'une seconde*. By soliciting that moment of surprise and estrangement from the ordinariness of cancer, the montage seeks to address its invisible presence in someone's life rather than its cellular claims on their body. Here too, as in Clara's double portrait, the narrative relation between the before and the after is still ablative. Something has been removed that otherwise eludes (clinical) representations of cancer (Fig. 5.4).

In response to the thought of cancer incidence, recording artist Stromae (Paul van Haver) generated a lyric proximate in the form of a quasi-homophonic question: "Quand c'est?" (2015).

> *Cancer, cancer, dis-moi quand c'est ?*
> *Cancer, cancer, qui est le prochain ?*
> (Cancer, cancer, tell me when?
> Cancer, cancer, who's next?).

In the song, *cancer* /kɑ̃.sɛʁ/ occupies the space vacated by the unanswered question (*quand c'est?* /kɑ̃/sɛ/). Visually, it is rendered as a monstrous shadow reminiscent of the allegorical cancer in mid-century French *affiches*, absent at first, then stealth and discreet, and finally overwhelming in the second half of the music video. "Cancer" takes over the entire theater—stage, seats, and screen, no longer as a shadow but as computer generated growths. That the totality of cancer understood as a total social fact (Jain 2013) should take a digital form was to be expected.

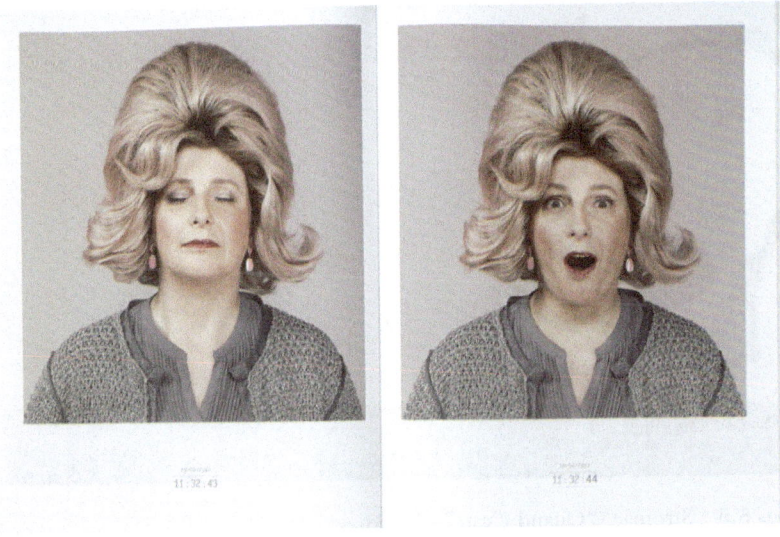

Fig. 5.4 Mimi Fondation, *Ne serait-ce qu'une seconde* (2013)

Stromae's mode of address turns the totality of cancer into familiarity ("We know each other quite well, don't we?"), familiarity into proximity (who's next?), and with the music video realized by Luc Van Haver (Stromae's brother) and Xavier Reyé, proximity into a choreography. The choreography may be a spatial rendition of the structure of address but it is also a modern take on the late Gothic theme of the *danse macabre*; only instead of skeletons and partially decomposed corpses leading the livings along, the articulated legs of a monstrous insect taunt Stromae's tall and slender silhouette. The dance is not macabre because it ends with the demise of the dancing silhouette. It is macabre because by the second half of the twentieth century, cancer had become, according to Philippe Ariès (1975, 173), the new image of death in the West (Figs. 5.5 and 5.6).

Not unlike poems calling upon the coreless ubiquity of the wind or the sky to be their rhetorical witness, *Quand c'est?* doesn't exactly put faces on cancer. Rather, the twinned questions "When?" and "Who's next?" fashion a series of silhouettes out of demographic entities: women and breast cancer ("you wanted to have my mother"), men and lung cancer ("And my father's lungs, do you remember them?"), and unspecified

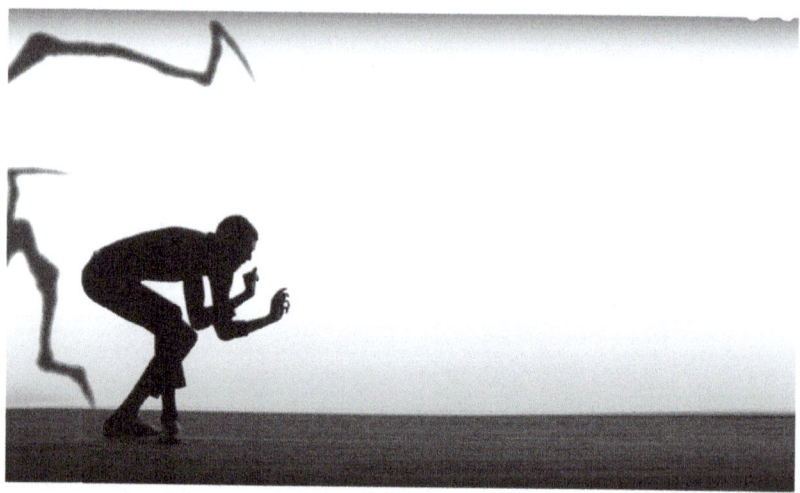

Fig. 5.5 Stromae, "Quand c'est?" (2013)

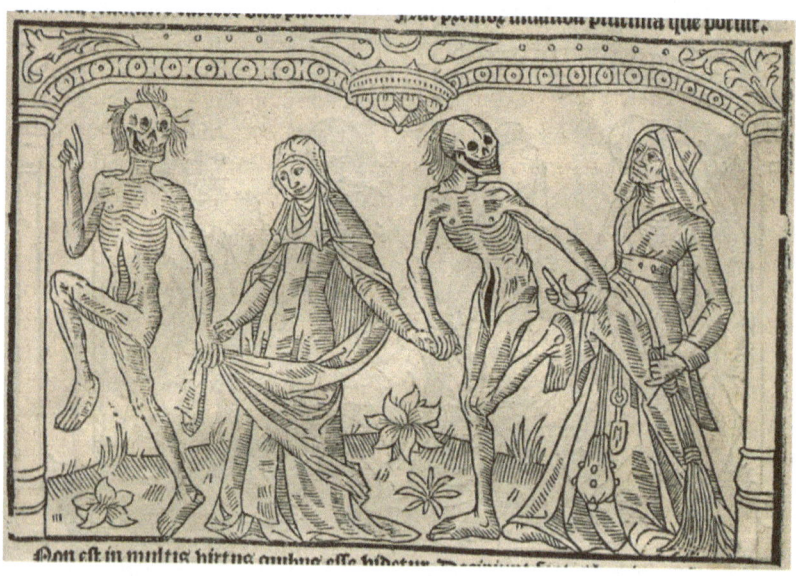

Fig. 5.6 Nicolas Le Rouge, *La grant danse macabre des hommes et des femmes hystoriée et augmentée de beaulx ditz en latin* (1528) (Courtesy Bibliothèque Municipale de Lille)

childhood cancer ("You like little children"). Epidemiology gives us reassurance that we belong in tangible and yet invisible ways to a population even though most of the time members of a population are left with little to no choice in the matter of their belonging.

CHAPTER 6

In the Meantime (*120 Beats Per Minute* 2017)

Abstract Robin Campillo's *120 Beats Per Minute* (2017) is the fast-paced chronicle of a time of transition toward a new therapeutic status quo for people with AIDS that never seems to arrive fast enough. It is a period piece directed some thirty years after futurity showed up in the form of protease inhibitors turning a terminal diagnosis into a medicated condition. The movie takes up residence on the narrow edge of a meantime that drains immunocompromised bodies waiting for a better course of treatment. Vignette 6 seeks to reoccupy this temporality from the perspective of epidemiological realism.

Keywords *120 Beats Per Minute* (film) · Activism · Campillo, Robin · Dance · HIV/AIDS · Terminality

Whether we want it or not, we live in an epidemiological reality made of statistical correlations (between wildfire smoke, reduced economic productivity, and eye cancer), risk factors and social determinants of health, animal reservoirs and spillovers, containment strategies and curves to be flattened, prophylactic measures, and syndromic surveillance systems detecting in real-time potential outbreaks. In fact, we have been living in an epidemiological reality for quite some time now, even before the formalization of epidemiological tools and concepts at the beginning of the twentieth century. Comparing medieval episodes of pestilence that inspired spectacular movements of public devotion to the societal impact of the epidemy of cholera in 1832, French conservative chronicler Chateaubriand was already putting his finder on something that felt like a shift toward the epidemiological present, when he wrote that "cholera reached us in a century of philanthropy, incredulity, newspapers, and material administration" (Cited in Huet 2012, 1). The claim that we live in an epidemiological reality, however, is not historical, at least not in the sense that it debates chronologies and chains of action, tracks down precedents, and identifies lessons that ought to be learned. If anything, as Christos Lynteris (2020) observed pointedly, "Global Health narratives are saturated by pronouncement of and reflections on 'the lessons of this' or 'the lessons of that' historical outbreak"—with little regard for what happens in the meantime.

Robin Campillo's *120 Beats Per Minute* (2017) is the fast-paced chronicle of a time of transition toward a new therapeutic status quo for people with AIDS that never seems to arrive fast enough. It is a period piece directed some thirty years after futurity showed up in the form of protease inhibitors turning a terminal diagnosis into a medicated condition. The movie takes up residence on the narrow edge of a meantime that drains immunocompromised bodies waiting for a better course of treatment. Its end point is not a triumphal entry into chronic time but Sean's death, a member of ACT UP Paris, and the grief of his friends, lovers, and fellow activists. It is not the chemical ever after of retroviral drugs but an ambiguous scene of protest to which I will return later.

BPM accounts for the deliberations of a group in the process of negotiating difficult coalitions and the difference between not enough and too much in an effort to stay true to a commitment to being deliberative even when the clock is ticking. Meetings can't go on forever. It's already too late for former members. It's already getting late for others. T-cell clocks are ticking. And yet, the film also chooses to linger on what seems peripheral to its immediate concerns and out of steps with the sense of urgency that drives everything else: plotting public interventions, testing out recipes for social impact, storming pharmaceutical labs, flirting, falling in and out of love, getting sick, going to the hospital, and dying.

I am drawn to these moments where the movie is getting long and breaks into dance, not unlike the characters in a musical. Clubbing sequences correspond to moments of optical shiftiness focusing on the

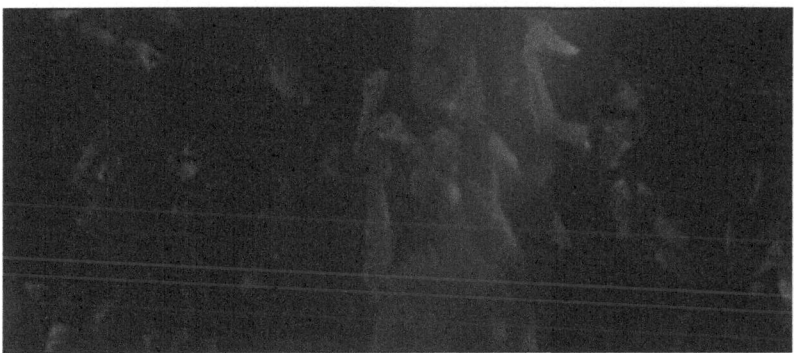

Fig. 6.1   First clubbing sequence. *120 battements par minute*

darkened space between the dancing bodies. There is something in the air that becomes visible as silhouettes throb and fade into the background suggesting an airborne event that does not make epidemiological sense in a movie about the AIDS crisis. Unless *BPM* itself is the airborne event: an exercise in raising the metaphorical dust that settled a generation ago on the other side of terminal time. Is the dustiness of the air an image of dirtiness, a marker of dangers that is all over the place (as opposed to out of place as in Mary Douglas)? (Bourdeau 2022). The particles in suspension take over the dancefloor unbeknownst to the dancers, erasing their contours to become cells attacked by a virus under a microscope. The shift from the dancing bodies to the dancing cells stands for the infinite distance between the dancing bodies and the viral ballet. And yet that distance is never so infinite that bodies don't get sick, infect each other, and when treatment is either not available or no longer tolerated, waste away (Figs. 6.1, 6.2 and 6.3).

Soon enough, the cellular ballet is over, replaced by the flatness of a drawing on a projected slide reflecting its light on worried faces and slouching bodies. The mesmerizing but deadly choreography of viral replication makes way for a highly technical theater of molecular intervention describing the therapeutic promises of protease inhibitors. The passage from the clubbing sequence to the biology lesson is yet another exercise in visualizing moments of inconsequential overlap between different versions of the body—"the body of anatomists and physiologists, the one science sees or discusses" and "a body of bliss consisting

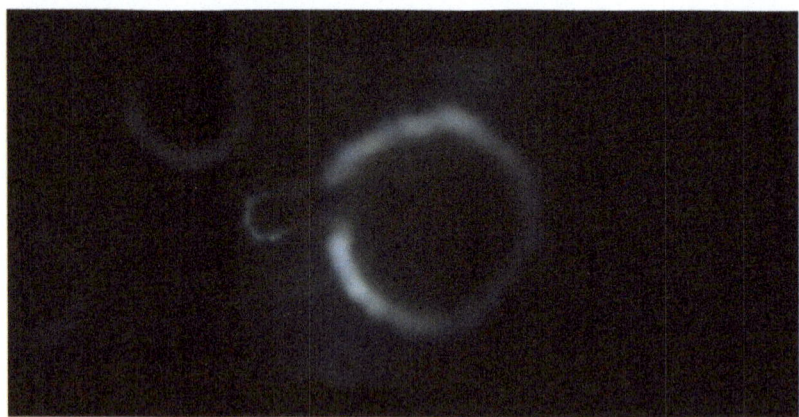

Fig. 6.2 First clubbing sequence. *120 battements par minute*

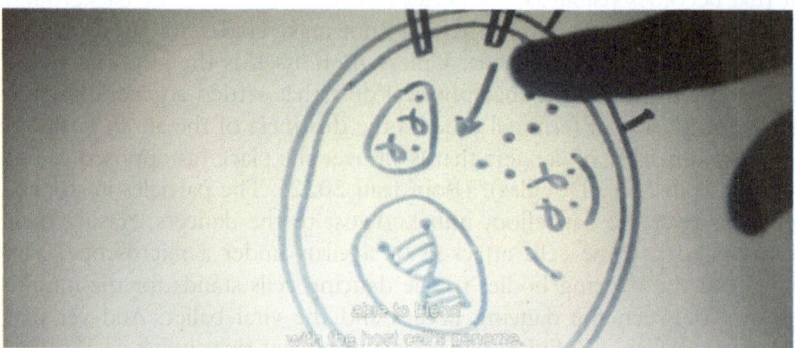

Fig. 6.3 Protease inhibitors slide. *120 battements par minute*

solely of erotic relations" (1975, 16). It is one thing to visualize a virus and the process through which it spreads in the body. It is another to visualize how physiological relations of causalities have social consequences. With its visuality out of joint, the initial clubbing sequence in *BPM* occupies in cinematographic terms the allegorical space of pestilence in a fifteenth-century Sienese book cover attributed to Giovanni di Paolo. It is tempting to understand this Biccherna image as the admonitory representation of an epidemiological event by non-epidemiological means. The

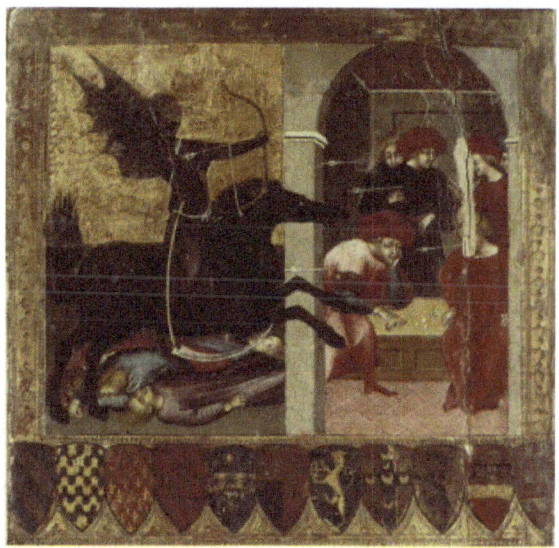

Fig. 6.4 Giovanni di Paolo, Biccherna book cover attributed to Giovanni di Paolo. Siena, Italy, 1437. poplar wood, tempera painting. 43 × 28 cm. Kunstgewerbemuseum, Staatliche Museen, Berlin, Germany (Photo Credit: bpk Bildagentur, Art Resource, NY)

arrows targeting the necks and the armpits—the seat of symptoms for the bubonic plague—suggest an unidentified relation of causality suspended in time. But if the winged silhouette on a black horse trampling the dead and assailing the still living contaminate and infect, it also distributes death at a distance before death was available to statistical capture in terms of frequency. It distributes death in painting, that is, in the same visual space where invisible entities manifest themselves in angelic forms in Fra Angelico's annunciations to administer the mystery of incarnation. Here the allegory of the plague is less an attempt to make the invisible visible than to locate invisible relations within a visual field (Fig. 6.4).

The clubbing sequences punctuating the movie are not simply moments of ecstatic relief in the midst of tensed verbal and physical exchange. Their strange lyricism is another expression of the AIDS crisis that, at the time of his involvement in ACT UP Paris, the future director of *BPM* also experienced as a visual enigma.[1] In an interview with Didier Péron, Campillo explains that the *cinema d'auteur* he admired as a film student seemed out of touch with an "event that was still difficult to recognize and that was generating names and images entirely foreign to [him]":

> names like Western Blot [an immunoassay technique] or Elisa test, the first apparition of the patients defaced by symptoms the disease, like Kenny Ramsauer as seen in a documentary that aired on ABC in 1983, and whose tragic birthday photographs taken with his boyfriend are reprinted in an issue of *Paris Match*. Art cinema is swept aside by the images that are starting to circulate during this time and that call to mind some kind of sci-fi flick about a spectacular and insidious disaster. (Campillo and Péron 2017)

The delay between the events depicted in *BPM* and the release of the film is thus not incidental to its subject matter. Cinema had to wait. For Campillo, futurity also shows up in the form of non-narrative moments of transition between action and deliberation, between dancing bodies and diseased bodies, between "electron microscopy or reconstructive computer graphics" and "a premodern vision of the body, according to which heresy and sin are held to be scored in their voluntary subjects by punitive and admonitory manifestations of disease" (Watney 1987, 78, 73). In them, the terminal temporality of HIV/AIDS achieves duration, a cinematic duration that, thanks to the entry of HIV/AIDS into chronic time, has the luxury of not being so onerous anymore.

BPM ends the way it started, with a scene of protest immediately followed by a short-lived clubbing sequence, so immediately in fact that it is as if one had morphed into the other. Only a few seconds before the end credits, the music stops before the dance does. Of course, there is nothing careless about this slight delay during which the sound of the dancers' steps on the dancefloor is no longer muffled by the soundtrack.

---

[1] Philippe Mangeot, president of Act Up-Paris from 1997 to 1999 and co-screenwriter of *120 BPM* with Campillo, comments: "If there is an enigma in the film, it is in the impossible articulation between the public stage—the weekly meetings—and the private one—the bedroom. Between the political body and the diseased body. The entire history of Act Up is situated at their seam—because the private is political, because the disease is a public matter. But this seam is not a superposition, and the stitching remains enigmatic" (Chémery et al. 2018, 114–115).

These few seconds of restlessness are the narrative equivalent of a quilting point that, on the one hand, channels the immersive feeling of time reenacted and held together by the magic of editing, while puncturing, on the other, the bitter promise of "a stainless world in which *we* will only be recalled in textbooks and carefully edited documentary 'evidence,' as signs of plagues and contagions averted" (Watney 1987, 86).

When I say restless, I have in mind a 2016 documentary on the end of the distinguished career of Wendy Wheelan, former principal dancer with the New York City Ballet. *Restless Creature* too is about a time of transition and the wisdom of endings. Wendy is thinking about retirement. But how can she retire as a dancer when dance for her is everything? It is her life, in a manner of speaking, although she is heard saying: "At times, I've thought if I don't dance, I'd rather die" without seeming literal enough for the macabre thought to cause concern. In a less dramatic register, Wendy hesitates between possible versions of an ending: the grand gesture or the subdued exit, so quiet nobody would notice, not even her. To cope with the distress and the uncertainty, she surrounds herself with the next generation of ballerinos and ballerinas. She meets with former colleagues who are still coming to terms with their own retirement and what it means to have retired a version of their body, and others who had to quit early. For Wendy, the prospects of retirement and the answer to the question of how to keep on dancing are tied to a torn ligament labrum injury, a surgery, and a painful rehabilitation process that turns the question on its head. How to end ballet? becomes Where does it end? Where does ballet end and where does physical rehabilitation begin? After all, if the Balanchine ballet is demanding so is physiotherapy. And no, physiotherapy is not choreography, but in *Restless Creature*, the two coexists in a *pas de deux*. One makes the other possible, or else, bearable. One repairs the damages caused by the other. But at any rate, how to tell physiotherapy and choreography apart if one cannot tell the dancer from the dance.

Restless Creature gives a literal "ring of urgency" (De Man 1977, 30) to the otherwise rhetorical question that concludes William Butler Yeats's poem. "Among School Children": "How can we know the dancer from the dance?" becomes "Please tell me, how *can* I know the dancer from the dance" (De Man 1977, 30) so I can keep on living. The distinction matters because by Wendy's own admission—"if I don't dance, I'd rather die"—the indifference to the distinction would amount to denying her an existence once the dance is over. Back to *BPM* restless creatures, the dancers from 1993 are not so different from the dancers in 2017. The difference is invisible—molecular really. 2017 dancers have access to life saving drugs. The carefully edited break in the soundtrack at the end of the movie sees the dancers through the moment of transition and delivers them safely on the other side of the transitional moment into the time of the chronic, where they can dance longer that they would have otherwise only a generation ago.

The terminal meantime *BPM* commemorates so vividly has come to pass, dissolving into what Eric Cazdyn (2012) describes as the new chronic: an age of ongoing crisis management that has moved away from a future organized by the belief in the possibility of a cure and a public health revolution. In an early twenty-first-century context where the U.S. government has put the public health legacy of the AIDS crisis to rest by dissolving the Presidential Advisory Council on HIV/AIDS and the Office of National AIDS Policy, the end of terminality also leaves us with things like the museification of David Wojnarowicz, an iconic figure from the Act Up movement, who died of the consequences of AIDS in 1992. In 2018, members of ACT UP-New York staged a silent protest of a Wojnarowicz retrospective at the Whitney Museum of American Art, handing and holding statements that read: "AIDS is not history. The AIDS crisis did not die with David Wojnarowicz." It may have come to a halt but it did not come to an end.

Campillo's gesture may be commemorative but *BPM* is not a resting place. In a way, it is akin to a belated action movie set in the heydays of the genre in the 1990s with *Die Hard* (1988), *Terminator II* (1991), *Speed* (1994), and *Armageddon* (1998). For Jameson (2003), the explosive frenzy of the 90 action movies is symptomatic of a widespread sense of temporal terminality borne by frantic bodies that are either always on the run and thus incapable of emotional depth, or too tired to keep going—and thus unable to sustain the narrative interest that the constant pyrotechnic drama demands from them. Hence the emphasis on closed loops: "a high-rise building, an airport, an airplane, a train, an elevator, or […] a city bus […] a whole city […] or indeed the earth itself as the meteor approaches" (Jameson 2003, 715). In *BPM*, the narrative closed loop is essentially demographic and generational. At some point, a biological time bomb that ticks to a T-cell countdown will go off in the night, off camera, without a bang but not without splatters of fake blood and a scattering of ashes turning a swanky corporate meeting into an angry funerary banquet.

CHAPTER 7

Statistical Interlude (Halbwachs 1913; Maupassant 1889)

Abstract In 1913, French sociologist Maurice Halbwachs was already putting his fingers on the fact that the distribution of mortality in a population could be understood as an indicator of whose social existence is fostered and whose is not. Lives are not just lived but administered. Going against the statistical model developed by Adolphe Quetelet, Halbwachs assigned a social systematicity to the frequency of variations. It means that statistics are not solely descriptive. They too tell a story. For Maupassant, this is more than a figure of speech but the premise of his short story "L'Endormeuse" (1889).

Keywords *120 Beats per Minutes* (film) · Halbwachs, Maurice · Maupssant, Guy · Life expectancy · Statistics

We are not quite done with *BPM*, Sean's death and his funeral arrangements, but first let's take a break and play *The Game of Life* a little with the help of the U.S. Social Security Administration (SSA) website. Just elect male or female then enter your age, the interface will do the rest. The result is straightforward, telling you how many years you have left to live and more importantly, for the purpose of the narrative exercise, to pay for from the time you are eligible to retire. This number is a rough

V. Bruyere, *Epidemiological Realism*, Palgrave Studies in Literature, Science and Medicine,
https://doi.org/10.1007/978-3-031-68517-0_7

53

approximation that doesn't take into account a long list of health determinants and predictive factors, such as preexisting conditions. The result can be straightforward because the machine has been designed to diminish the amount of narrative friction between past, present, and future in the system.

The plot is simple but the implications of this quick narrative exercise are life altering, especially if it is the first time that your mortality appears to you on a timeline. From now on, you may start believing in your own death. In fact, you better believe in it for it is the only way you will be able, not just to endure the life you live—in the words of Jacques Lacan (2017, 11)—but to survive your non-productive years. If believing proves itself to be too hard, there is also an app for that. WeCroak® was designed to rehearse with you what it feels to be mortal by reminding you of your death five times a day but without a specific timeline.

You may already know that populations have been statistical objects of inquiry for several centuries, but it does not automatically mean that you have a good grasp on what your statistical membership in a population entails in terms of responsibility and self-management, and how to draw the line between the statistical now and the actuarial future when fate can weigh in at any moment. Life expectancy, rather than fate, powers the SSA interface. Life expectancy represents a cluster of actual individuals within a birth cohort. It corresponds to the apex of a bell curve graph representing variations within a population at a certain moment of time (at birth, at age 5, at age 50… etc.). For life expectancy to be averaged out, all members of a cohort must have died. So in the meantime, and before a statistical value can be obtained, it will have to remain a probability based on a current estimate.

Perhaps the object of belief here is less the statistical image of your own death than the logics of accumulation and aggregation that power the SSA projection: the aggregation that yields an average value and the accumulation (of years and capital) that secures future benefits. If so, the narrative exercise starts to look like an adult version of the Stanford marshmallow experiment: a behavioral experiment designed by Walter Mischel and his team in the 1960s and 1970s with the objective of finding evidence of a correlation between the ability to wait for delayed gratification and later success in life. The experiment involved a feeding mechanism and children left in a room for variable periods of time with a treat (such as a marshmallow) in front of them. They can eat the marshmallow now or have it twice later if they are patient enough and wait for the return of the adult in charge—or, as Lochlan Jain puts it, if they have enough trust in the rewarding structure and its figures of authority (2013, 57). In the meantime, the world might end, or the reserve of treats could run dry. Worse even, the incentive itself could lose its appeal.

The worst-case scenario becomes the norm in a health system where "the poor and less poor are less likely to live long enough to enjoy the good life whose promise is a fantasy bribe that justifies so much exploitation" (Berlant 2011, 105). Povinelli (2006, 54–56) offers a variation on what this scenario looks like in her work on the reproduction of Aboriginal life in northwest Australia. It corresponds to a situation in which the political recognition and the continuing existence of a vulnerable community is made to depend on the testimony and memory of elders in that same community at a moment of demographic transition where the life expectancy within this group is such that it may not allow some of its members to grow old enough to become agents of recognition before the State.

In 1913, Maurice Halbwachs was already putting his finger on the fact that the distribution of mortality in a population could be understood as an indicator of whose social existence is fostered and whose is not. Lives are not just lived until the candle is spent or the wicker snuffed, but administered. Going against the statistical model developed by Adolphe Quetelet, according to which, for human variations to be represented in a bell curve, one had to consider the distribution of values within a population as random or non-assignable, Halbwachs assigned a social systematicity to the frequency of variations (Canguilhem 1991, 161). This is why, he explained, "a society has, in general, the mortality that suits it, and that the number of deaths and their distribution across different age groups aptly expresses the importance attached by society to the fact that life could be more or less prolonged" (1913, 97). It also means that statistics are not solely descriptive. They tally but they too tell a story.[1]

For Maupassant, this is more than a figure of speech. The debate over the descriptive power of statistics forms the premise of another short story. *L'Endormeuse*—literally "The Sleep Inducer," or more apropos, "The Sleep Machine"—first published in the columns of *L'Écho de Paris* on September 16, 1889, paints a gruesome tableau of social suffering:

---

[1] On the tension between tallying and telling, see, for instance, the reading of Daniel Defoe's *Journal of the Plague Year* (1722) in Weber (2022, 107–121).

In the first paper I opened I noticed this headline, "Statistics of Suicides," and I read that more than 8,500 persons had killed themselves in that year. In a moment I seemed to see them! [...] I saw men bleeding, their jaws fractured, their skulls cloven, their breasts pierced by a bullet, slowly dying, alone in a little room in a hotel, giving no thought to their wound, but thinking only of their misfortunes. (Maupassant 1922, 1)

For the nameless narrator, numbers are not abstractions but unbearable images assailing him. The statistical scattering of death is felt with such intensity that it triggers a daydream set five years into a dystopian future where a non-profit organization—"The Foundation for Voluntary Death"—has taken upon itself to address the suicide epidemic. The secretary of the foundation understands suicide as a social inconvenience—an eyesore in an otherwise spotless bourgeois décor, something unfortunate but unavoidable in dire need of rebranding.

The centerpiece of the centralized program is the eponymous sleep machine: a chaise lounge, luxuriously outfitted, divan-like, and designed as if it had been made for talking and listening but discretely equipped to vaporize death in the form of an inodorous gas that can be perfumed ad libitum. The gassing chair functions like a reverse hot-line of sort. It *administers* death in both sense of the term: it delivers death painlessly as a solution to social suffering and regulates its representation. Death is to be rendered painless but so too its representation. There will be no more gruesome mental tableaus formed in the narrator's mind. "Death need not be sad," the secretary explains, "it should be a matter of indifference." By representing death as a state of indifference, "the sleeping machine" creates conditions in which numerical values can in effect capture social relations (from birth to death). It is also in that sense that death is administered in the numbing face of incidence.

Maupassant's short story offers a striking version of what of Kathleen Woodward (1999) called "statistical panic" intuiting the unchecked power of numbers in the governance of human affairs. *L'Endormeuse* version of statistical panic comes from a time where the substitution between bodies and numbers was not fully automated yet. Hence perhaps the dream of the machine. Mary Beth Mader goes a step further in her characterization of the quantitative capture of social relations by assimilating the statistical "distribution of mortality risk [...] to the commemorative ritual of ashes scattering" (2012, 65). To be clear, the analogy is not between two substances—ashes and statistics—but between two memorial gestures: ash-scattering and statistical capture (and the release of data). That said, the parallel drawn here between a substance and an abstraction also reads as an invitation to substantiate statistics.

The terms of a reverse scenario turning ashes into numerical ratios are being explored toward the end of *BPM* when members of ACT UP Paris try to negotiate with Sean's mother what percentage of her son's ashes she intends to keep and how much they will be able to devote to the political funeral he wanted. Are we talking 50/50, 40/60, or more like 80/20? The negotiation is not tense, just awkward. Its outcome remains undisclosed but not unresolved since the political funeral will eventually take place and return Sean's public persona to the scene of his activism by scattering what's left of him on trays of dainty canapés during a health insurance convention. No matter how much or how little of her son's ashes the mother will have agreed to let go, the division of Sean's two bodies is already a scene of scattering that leaves something of him suspended, in suspension.

CHAPTER 8

Occupational Realism (*Severance* 2018)

Abstract In Ling Ma 2018 debut novel *Severance*, the world comes to an end without first coming to a halt. Shen fever has created something like a postural limbo, where fevered subjects rehearse endlessly everyday gestures and habits until their zombified body has been fully consumed by them, allowing infrastructures to collapse while crisis ordinariness endures. The horror is cautiously allegorical: if crisis ordinariness doesn't lead to revolutionary action or at least something collective and aspirational, it is because Shen fever infected a world where work, the division of labor, and an all-encompassing supply chain are the main forms under which collective existence—and, conversely, a biographical sense of self-worth—is both organized and valued. It is that element in Ma's script that achieved an anticipatory status in March 2020.

Keywords Pandemic extinction · Pneumoconiosis · *Severance* (novel) · Work conditions · Zola, Emile · Zombies

In *Modernity at large*, Arjun Appadurai points out that "we live in a world of many kinds of realism, some magical, some socialist, some capitalist, and some that are yet to be named" (1996, 54). There is the realism that "establishes imagined communities, teaches people how to

© The Author(s), under exclusive license to Springer Nature 59
Switzerland AG 2024
V. Bruyere, *Epidemiological Realism*, Palgrave Studies in Literature,
Science and Medicine,
https://doi.org/10.1007/978-3-031-68517-0_8

think about the world as the product of shared spatial and temporal logics, and reinforces the sense that any narrative takes place against the backdrop of an ongoing historical and geographic structure that functions [...] relatively independently of the activity of any given story" (Hayot 2012, 124). There is the end of that realism in a world shaken by superstorms and inhabited by climate refugees (Gosh 2016). And there is the epidemiological realism that "train[s] entire nations of viewers to imagine the presence of invisible pathogens in scenarios of consumption and exchange" (Ostherr 2005, 3). Appadurai connects the proliferation of realisms to the fact that more and more people across the world invest their world with prospects of a different life. It does not mean that the world is a better place where everyone gets to live the life they want, only that even "the harshest of lived inequalities are now open to the play of the imagination" (1996, 54). For Rancière (2017b), this is indeed what the realism of Flaubert is about. His novels and novellas went to great stylistic lengths to extend the power of fantasy to a new class of fictional characters that until then had been excluded from the realm of romance and affective excess.

In her debut novel, *Severance* (2018), Ling Ma tells the story of how Candace Chen shelved her fantasy of becoming a photographer in the steps of Nan Goldin to instead work an office job at a big publishing company in New York City. She is in charge of choreographing the many moving parts of the supply chain behind the production of bibles of all kinds (bejeweled, affordable, customizable... etc.). It's not the career she dreamed of or studied for, but it's work; it's better than nothing, and she is rather good at what she does. *Severance* also happens to be the story of a pandemic apocalypse set in an alternative version of 2011. The outbreak of Shen fever, a fictional disease named after Shenzhen, in southeastern China, where the airborne disease caused by fungal spores originated, is uncontained, unstoppable, and incurable. If in the uplifting words of novelist Arundhati Roy in early April 2020, pandemics are agents of historical transformations, "portal[s] [...] between one world and the next," *Severance*, by contrast, stages a catastrophic crisis of planetary proportions without seizing the opportunity to go wild with the revolutionary possibilities a post-apocalyptic world would be susceptible to offer (to torch everything, to take charge, to be heroic, to start fresh, to dream big at last). Instead, the novel develops a first-person satirical thought experiment, almost surgical in its detached and witful narrative delivery, dwelling on the absence of radical difference between the two versions of the world, before and after the outbreak. Even the distinction between healthy and infected bodies is thin in the early stage of the disease.[1]

Throughout the novel and starting with the opening sentence—"After the End came the Beginning" (Ma 2018, 3)—the back and forth between now—after the world ended—and then—just before the End—is less a study in contrasts than in symmetries between civilization and its post-apocalyptic afterlives. Survivalism, for instance, is hardly the stuff of fantasy in Ma's novel. Not only it has been already all played out by mainstream culture, but it also a lot of tedious work that relies heavily on routinization anchored in a strict division of labor. In the same way that the bohemian drift her boyfriend embraces doesn't appeal to Candace, the survivalist scenario does not work for her the way it worked for Bob—the mid-level manager turned militia figurehead and charismatic leader—by giving him the world he always wanted.[2]

In *Severance*, the world comes to an end without first coming to a halt. Shen fever has created something like a postural limbo, where fevered subjects rehearse endlessly everyday gestures and habits until their zombified body has been fully consumed by them, allowing infrastructures to collapse while crisis ordinariness endures. The horror is cautiously allegorical: if civilizational collapse does not lead to revolutionary action or doesn't translate into something collective and aspirational, it is because Shen fever infected a world where work, the division of labor, and an all-encompassing supply chain are the main forms under which collective existence—and, conversely, a biographical sense of self-worth and purpose—is both organized and expressed. It is that element in Ma's script that achieved an anticipatory status in March 2020. If Flaubertian realism, Rancière (2017, 15) explains in his rereading of *A Simple Heart*, was about what it meant for a dutiful servant, a model of work ethics, to be capable of "going to the most extreme lengths of physical and moral

---

[1] Dora Zhang (2020) describes the tone as "hovering between non-contempt and non-endorsement." On the ambiguous and potentially compromised status of the narrator, see Yazell and Hsu (2020, 40): "At various moments, the novel invites us to question whether Candace herself is infected: what is the difference between this drive to lose herself in work routines and the fevered repetitions of time-loop zombies."

[2] The blurring between before and after, between civilization and its afterlife is also available to the novel in a ritualized form when Candace burns fake money and images of luxury goods cut from magazines in an offering to her deceased parents. See Ma (2018, 104).

degradation in order to satisfy her passions," COVID realism was about who is capable of reworking their relation to work on the spot, to keep on working, to work remotely, and who is not.

In the conclusion of his ethnography of avian influenza in Hong Kong, Keck argues that the claim of pandemic narratives to totality emerged toward the end of the twentieth century as a counter-response to the form of social totality claimed at the beginning of the twentieth century by proletarian theories of the general strike that would bring the world of production and transactions to a halt. The hypothesis of a pandemic imaginary with a classist agenda that "represent[s] the cessation of global activity as an eventuality for which [a new bourgeoisie] has been preparing itself" (Keck 2010, 295) while concepts of strike and working class lost some of their initial mobilizing power is provocative.[3] It takes epidemiological realism back to the realist question of what it means to be capable of fantasy, to dare dreaming of a different life, to want a world instead of just being stuck with one. According to the critical diagnosis ran by Cazdyn (2012, 202), the aggressive zombie scenario—*28 Days Later*, *The Walking Dead*—belongs to a world in which the idea of the nation state remains the mode of organization of collective existence. In this scenario, the nation state is either gone, in ruins, or on the brink but remains the point of reference. The compliant compulsive zombies—or "time loop zombie"—of *Severance* belong to a world in which work, whether waged or unwaged, gainful or injurious, is the primary social form organizing collective existence. The habitual life of the fevered is what's left of collective existence after the demise of social literacy. It seems allegorically fitting then that the Shen fever outbreak would find its origin in the toxic atmosphere of a manufacturing hub in a special economic zone (SEZ) rather than in the sudden clash of worlds (the wet market and the metropolis) and tenses (the modern and the backward) as it is usually the case in the world of xenophobic outbreak narratives.[4]

You could say Ma's realism is bleak: she imagines the flaccid end of global capitalism but fails or refuses to dissociate it from the end of the world, which means that we are stuck with it. There is no world left to inhabit in absence of an extractivist and capitalist script that contributed

---

[3] In the COVID context, Paul Preciado (2020) pitched his argument about the de-collectivizing dimension of confinement in the vicinity of a comparable hypothesis.

[4] On the medical "nativist model" pitting the primordial against the modern and its role in the shaping of the SARS outbreak narrative see Wald (2008, 6–9).

to the emergence of the spores causing Shen fever. In that respect, it is bleak when it could have been both cautionary and relatable on an anticipatory mode as a future to be held in abeyance. But Ma's realism is also essentially anthropological to the extent that, in Lynteris's argument (2019), pandemic scenarios of human extinction are less about the odds of biological survival than what it means to be human after mastery—that is, to be human in relation to a world that has never been mastered after all because it was beyond mastery to start with.

You could also say *Severance* realism is occupational in a strong sense that Ma hints at in an interview with Jennifer Mills (2018):

> I don't think it's possible to break from capitalism. That is the world we live in. And I don't think writers should try to separate themselves from the world. We should all take jobs as stockbrokers, real estate agents, accountants—not just because that's how a lot of people live. In order to address the problem or even figure out what the problem is, we should spend time within the system, we should understand how the mechanics work. We should understand what it's like to hold down a soul-sucking position, the personal stakes and fears associated with that—but also, what it's like to be seduced by a job that you don't believe in, that has moral ambiguities.[5]

Candace stays behind to staff the editorial office when anybody else has left the city in exchange for a large but ultimately undisclosed amount of money. The amount doesn't matter in the end, because the money has no market value in the absence of a market. There is nothing left to buy. Property and goods are now to be claimed and looted, not traded or purchased. At that point of the novel, Candace work ethics has been purified from its wage-earning purpose. All that is left is a feeling that too, sooner or later, fades away. Like the previews of humanity in its fossil state painted by Alan Weisman in *The World Without Us* (2007), *Severance* is a thought experiment: "Suppose that the worst has happened. Human extinction is a fait accompli" (2007, 4), how does one stay with the thought of a world we are left to inhabit on impossible terms? Or in Candace's version: what do you show up for when you are still showing up to work after the world has ended?

---

[5] On realism as an observational mode of facing up to the density of the world rather than as complicit mode of habituation to the status quo see Love (2016).

It is with Ma's occupational apocalypse in mind that I revisit the dialogue between Etienne and Bonnemort at the beginning of Émile Zola's coal mining novel *Germinal* (1885). In the opening pages of the novel, the object-scene of Zola's occupational realism is a dying body that keeps on living:

> – […] I caught a cold a month ago. I never used to cough; now I can't get rid of it. And the weird thing is that I spit, that I spit…"
> The rasping was again heard in his throat, followed by the black expectoration.
> – Is it blood? asked Etienne, daring, finally, to question him.
> Bonnemort slowly wiped his mouth with the back of his hand.
> – It's coal. I've got enough in my carcass to warm me till the end of my days. And it's five years since I put a foot down below. I stored it up, it seems, without knowing it; well, it embalms! (1894, 6–7. Modified translation)

In that scene, coal—or rather pneumoconiosis[6]—kills a miner while keeping him alive enough to tell the story of what it means to live or have lived a miner's life. It is at once inside and outside, inert and active, organic ("Is it blood?") and mineral ("It's coal"), at once in the background as a totalizing principle and at the forefront of the narrative development as an overwhelming non-human clamor seeping through the dialogue it interrupts.

Even though he has been marked for death from the outset—his name translates literally as "Good Death," almost as a greeting ("Good night!")—Bonnemort gets to live on until the end of the novel, unlike the other miners who drowned, were buried alive, or shot by the police. He is still alive but in an uncertain biographical state: in extreme poverty, strapped to a chair, barely sentient, by all accounts more still life than portrait. That is until his shadowy stillness seizes an allegorical opportunity in presence of Cécile Grégoire, the daughter of one of the coalmine principal shareholders:

> Gradually Bonnemort seemed to awake, he perceived her and examined her in his turn. A flame mounted to his cheeks, a nervous spasm drew his mouth, from which flowed a thin streak of black saliva. Fascinated, they

---

[6] Against all odds, the term "pneumoconiosis"—"an umbrella term for a group of lung diseases" caused by the inhalation of dust—is featured in *Severance* (2018, 24).

remained opposite each other—she flourishing, plump, and fresh from the long idleness and sated comfort of her race; he swollen with water, with the pitiful ugliness of a foundered beast, destroyed from father to son by a century of work and hunger. [...]

It was never possible to establish the exact facts. Why had Cécile come near? How could Bonnemort, nailed to his chair, have been able to seize her throat? [...] It seemed to be an outbreak of sudden madness [*un coup brusque de démence*], a longing to murder before this white young neck. Such savagery was stupefying in an old invalid, who had lived like a worthy man, an obedient brute, opposed to new ideas. What rancour, unknown to himself, by some slow process of poisoning, had risen from his bowels to his brain? The horror of it led to the conclusion that he was unconscious, that it was the crime of an idiot. (Zola 1894, 441)

An outbreak narrative can be the beginning of something new and emancipatory. It has the potential to outlast its initial claims to crisis. Or it can also be just that: a storytelling exercise, an episode, perhaps a temporary escape from the pressure of a system that can only be reformed by an apocalyptic scenario, and a cautionary move to reinvest everything there is to hope for in stifling scripts of a return to (what felt) normal. In the translation of the noted British sexologist Havelock Ellis, Zola's "outbreak of madness" is precisely the kind of threading disparaged by Georg Lukács: "The so-called action is only a thread on which the still lives are disposed in a superficial, ineffective fortuitous sequence of isolated, static pictures" (1971, 144). The epidemiological realism of the scene defies explanation and disarms the keenest observer. It is out of sequence and somewhat gratuitous but also somewhat anticipatory. It already occupies the space of zombie horror.

CHAPTER 9

Occupational Realism II (Mold Horror)

Abstract Mold seems to be having a moment in the register of horror at the beginning of the twenty-first century. Dust had its time as an emerging object of epidemiological concern at the end of the nineteenth century. Dust and mold may not be that different from an epidemiological perspective but the distinction this vignette entertains is primarily aesthetic. Dust and mold carry different association. Dust is archival, at once a deposit and a concentrate of reality—of the kind of reality, that is, history is supposed to be made of. Moldy continuity doesn't avail itself to historical time.

Keywords Dust · Black mold · Moldiness · Flaubert, Gustave · Foucault, Michel · Horror · Jameson, Fredric · Occupational medicine

Epidemiological realism leans toward horror. Or is it horror that leans toward epidemiology? There's nothing too surprising about that mutual attraction in the present if one follows Altschuler's argument about the gothic genealogy of global health in the nineteenth century and the idea that "the gothic [...] provided a form for narrating how unseen and frightening elements could infiltrate familiar spaces" (2017, 570). Mold seems to be having a moment in the register of horror at the beginning of the twenty-first century. Dust had its time as an emerging object of epidemiological concern at the end of the nineteenth century. Dust and mold may not be that different from an epidemiological perspective but the distinction I entertain here is primarily aesthetic.

Dust and mold carry different association. Dust is archival, at once a deposit and a concentrate of reality—of the kind of reality, that is, history is supposed to be made of. It is the stuff of historians and their calling. "Dust," Carolyn Steedman writes, is what "allowed [Jules Michelet] a perception of time as a kind of seamless duration in which past and future could not be sundered" (Steedman 2002, 161). The dust of factuality ("*la poussière des faits*"), according to a critical review of *Discipline and Punish*, is precisely what's missing in Michel Foucault's "cloudy" argument about the reform of the penitentiary system (Léonard 1980). But the cloud metaphor doesn't get us far enough. Let's say then that mold horror, not unlike Foucault's argument in *Discipline and Punish* (1977), seeks to "demystify what stands for the real understood as a totality that needs to be restituted. There's no such thing as 'the' real one reaches, provided one takes everything into account or certain things that are more 'real' than others, and that one fails to reach when focusing instead on fleeting abstractions" (Foucault 1994, 15).[1] Moldy continuity doesn't avail itself to historical time, in part because, compared to dust, it sticks too much to surfaces and is less easily set aside, contained, or washed away. Which is also why mold horror could be having its moment as a possible—if unwelcomed—narrative development in that thing literary scholars call realism.

To be sure, in the context of horror cinema, black mold is no less metaphorical than Michelet's dust. It vaporizes—as opposed to dissipates—the horror of geriatric dementia in *Relic* (Natalie Erika James 2020), a vague childhood trauma in *Black Mold* (John Pata 2023), femicidal violence in *The Haunting of Hill House* (Mike Flanagan 2018), or even, in Dawn Keetley's (2021) interpretation of mold horror, the fear of white extinction. In the horror register, black mold is a form that lends specificity to (the) pervasiveness (of ageism and racism). At a basic visual

---

[1] Likewise, there is such thing as an epidemiological reality, because "a type of rationality, a way of thinking, a program, a technique, a set of rational and coordinated efforts, objectives that are both defined and pursued, instruments to achieve it, etc., all this is real even if it does not claim to be "reality" itself nor "the" entire society" (Foucault 1994, 15).

level, it forms patches, sometimes a trail. In time, the patch spreads and comes to define a surface (wall, ceiling, staircase) and redefine an entire volume as cursed or nefarious. It is in that sense that mold horror is an invitation "to think architecturally about realism" (Kornbluh 2015, 199). To think realism architecturally is to posit that realism does more than bear witness to the unravelling of a world—for instance, the *ancien régime* in the context of French nineteenth-century realism—but indeed takes part in the construction of whatever comes after in the ruins of history. The moldy walls and atmospherics that a certain strain of horror seems to be favoring bring us back to the threshold of Madame Aubain moldy sitting room in Flaubert *A Simple Heart* and Jameson's key reading of that moldiness as a textual event.

Moldiness avails itself to epidemiology. It can be tracked. It has a source and thus belongs de facto to the secular world of cause and effect—even if from an epidemiological perspective there is a lack of evidence correlating toxic mold syndrome and the spores of *Stachybotrys chartarum* (Borchers et al. 2017). There is a reasonable hygrometric explanation for the moldy smell of Madam Aubain sitting room to be found in the difference of level between inside and outside: "The whole room smelt a little moldy [*moisi*] as [*car*] the floor was on lower level than the garden." And yet, there is more to the ambient moldiness than a faulty folding in the gridding of the world where the garden meets the house. The tracking leads nowhere: either back to the open grid that situates the intersection between the inside and the outside at another intersection ("between an alley and a narrow street"), or else back to a disembodied sensor. According to Jameson "this is the only perceptual sentence in the entire description—the only one which flexes what survives of the older bodily sensorium, the only concrete practice of perception still feebly surviving in a new odourless and qualityless universe" (1985, 380). Meanwhile, in the same room, in the same paragraph, the famous barometer that hangs on the wall above the piano registers something in the air that cannot be smelled.

The still life with barometer on the piano is where Barthes (1968) locates the object-scene of Flaubert realism. The barometer is a prop—the kind of object that next to other objects of the like create the pleasure of the period piece, or in different circumstances, the forensic pleasures of figuring out the pieces of a puzzle. Barthes explains that realism had to justify that kind of descriptive expenditure. There is an implicit definition of realism there that is both formal and historical. Formal because it is understood as contract between narration and description. Historical because the reality effect is understood to be replacing *ekphrasis* as the justification for the descriptive expenditure. For Barthes, the barometer is exemplary because narrative analysis struggles to account for it. For Rancière (2017b) on the other hand, its exemplarity has to do with the diffuse historical sense that the description takes place in a time where what makes a plot a plot is from now on up in the air. The room smelt "a little moldy" but probably not enough to raise alarm and function as a gothic symptom. No mold horror awaits who dares to enter Flaubert's novella.

CHAPTER 10

Scenes of Plotlessness (Woolf 1926; Camus 1947)

Abstract In her 1926 essay "On Being Ill," Virginia Woolf reflects on the apparent disinterest of literature for the experience of illness and ventures that "the public would say that a novel devoted to influenza lacked plot." Vignette 10 explains how this plotlessness achieved a certain form of prescience in an age of syndromic surveillance where epidemics exist in a suspended diagnostic state as trending searches on Google, trending topics on social media platforms, spotted spikes of over-the-counter drugs sold in a given location, and mutually self-reinforcing feedback loops in real time. Real time is a state of plotlessness. The immediacy of syndromic surveillance is essentially associative.

Keywords Camus, Albert · Influenza · *Plague, the* (novel) · Syndromic surveillance · Woolf, Virginia

Jim: Do you know what I was thinking?
    Selena: You were thinking that you will never hear a piece of original music ever again. You'll never read a book that hasn't already been written or see a film that hasn't been shot. (Boyle 2002)

© The Author(s), under exclusive license to Springer Nature Switzerland AG 2024
V. Bruyere, *Epidemiological Realism*, Palgrave Studies in Literature, Science and Medicine,
https://doi.org/10.1007/978-3-031-68517-0_10

Because it is lodged inside a film, Danny Boyle's *28 Days Later* (2002), Selena's elegy for a world on its knees belies the position of safety from which we are receiving her thoughts about the zombie apocalypse she is trying to survive. No matter of how devastating the pandemic scenario and no matter how many scenarios we can come up with, the prospects of pandemic extinction they offer are always already dampened by their very existence as stories and the narrative achievement that they represent, even before representing apocalyptic states of disarray. This does not mean that pandemic extinction scenarios are systematically unrealistic. Only that we relate to them in the register of fantasy, as the fantasy of surviving oneself as the spectator of a movie that will have never been shot.

Virginia Woolf's essay "On Being Ill" (1926) was written in the wake of one of the most devastating pandemics in recorded history but do not expect to find flights of apocalyptic fancy in its pages. Instead, the tone is quietly inquisitive: Why has literature not paid more attention to illness? Why novels haven't been devoted to influenza? Woolf (1926, 33) ventures that "the public would say that a novel devoted to influenza lacked plot." It would, on the assumption that flu, whether seasonal or pandemic, brings the world to a halt and that bedridden bodies lack the energy it takes to plan conquest and engage in conspiracies. In that sense, a feverish disposition is a form of dispensation: reclining bodies are more suited to a poetic state of being than they are to the novel because of poetry's elective affinities with non-linear relations and scenes of an existence out of sequence. From Woolf's perspective as a novelist, influenza is less an epidemiological reality, than a bodily posture with narrative ramifications. It does not mean that influenza does not exist—or that it exists only as a feverish state of mind—but that it cannot exist in a realist universe because of the way its effect on the organism unravels the contours of reality. It is as if one had to be a modernist writer to devote a novel to influenza (Belling 2009). To wit, a novel devoted to influenza would lack in plot because it is likely to be filled with descriptions and moments of reveries. On the flipside, should it contemplate something like a pandemic extinction scenario, it will likely drive itself into a state of plotlessness— hence Elana Gomel's mirror statement (Gomel 2000, 409): "The plot of pestilence is driven toward narrative exhaustion."

It is not the first time that a conjectural public has indicted the prospects of a plotless novel—and it won't be the last. It's precisely the kind of charge that has been brought against the descriptive overindulgence of French realist novelists by a leftist critique looking for strong narrative directions in a world losing sight of social totalities. Ironically enough, similar charges were also brought by socially conservative commentators lamenting a state of affairs where everything goes and everybody gets to have a destiny and experience intense and destructive, passions irrespective of their given stations in life (Rancière 2017b). At any rate, the public's pronouncement about the plotlessness of a novel devoted to influenza channeled by Woolf's essay has achieved a certain form of prescience in an age of syndromic surveillance where epidemics exist in a suspended diagnostic state as trending searches on Google, trending topics on social media platforms, spotted spikes of over-the-counter drugs sold in a given location, and mutually self-reinforcing feedback loops.

Wherever the "public" has an internet connection, programs like "Sickweather" or "Flu detector" (also known as i-sense flu) track epidemic developments in real time (Caduff 2014, 43). Real time is a state of plotlessness. The immediacy of syndromic surveillance is essentially associative—as is this passage of a novel that Roland Barthes accused too of lacking plot[1]:

the word 'plague' [...] conjured up in the doctor's mind not only what science chose to put into it, but a whole series of fantastic possibilities utterly out of keeping with that gray and yellow town under his eyes [...] old pictures of the plague: Athens, a charnel-house reeking to heaven and deserted even by the birds; Chinese towns cluttered up with victims silent in their agony; the convicts at Marseille piling rotting corpses into pits; the building of the Great Wall in Provence to fend off the furious plague-wind; the damp putrefying pallets stuck to the mud floor at the Constantinople lazar-house, where the patients were hauled up from their beds with hooks, the carnival of masked doctors at the Black Death, men and women copulating in the cemeteries of Milan, cartloads of dead bodies rumbling through London's ghoul-haunted darkness—nights and days filled always, everywhere, with the eternal cry of human pain. (Camus 1991, 39–40)

Here Albert Camus mimics by anticipation the cascading effect that a word—plague—can have in a hyperlinked environment. The jumbled sequence of "old images" in the mind of the good doctor reads like the

---

1 "There is no structure to The Plague, no causes, no links between *The Plague* and an elsewhere that could be the past and other places, and other events" (Barthes 1991, 452).

result of a Google search, or, perhaps like the down-the-rabbit-hole effect induced by click baits taking you to an elsewhere that is only and always just another link away.

CHAPTER 11

Scenes of Contagion (Poussin, ca. 1630; Soderbergh 2011)

Abstract This vignette circulates between scenes of contagion in early modern visual culture and in Steven Soderbergh pandemic thriller *Contagion* (2011). When he paints touch and contagion, Nicolas Poussin gives us to see tears in the fabric of a social world. When Soderbergh films disembodied touch and cough, he alludes to the deceitfulness of surfaces and empty spaces that are never as innocent or clean as they seem to be, and thus to invisible modes of transmission.

Keywords *Contagion* (film) · Diagram · Emerging infectious diseases · Fomite · Girard · René · Pandemic thriller · *Plague of Ashdod, the* (painting) · Poussin, Nicolas · Zoonosis

Let's not close that window quite yet. If you keep on scrolling passed images of the Great Wall in Provence and the Constantinople lazar-house, you may find yourself in the virtual presence of Nicolas Poussin's *The Plague of Ashdod* (1628–1630), a spectacular painting that is very much out of its element in the COVID present. In her meticulous engagement with the painting, Sheila Barker tells us that "only once we suspend our contemporary conceptions of plague and human biology can we begin to reconstruct the range of medical issues that framed Poussin's enterprise during his own age" (2004, 659). In other words, the truth of the painting is in its historical context: Poussin paints the plague at a time where Robert Burton, among others, claimed that "the agitated imagination [could] kill" (Barker 2004, 660). The plague is not in the painting like it is under the microscope, in an animal reservoir, a zoonotic diagram, preserved as a specimen awaiting to be disposed of, or put to work in a lab setting. The pestilence that Poussin paints is to be understood primarily in narrative, affective, and visual terms within a context that has no use for liquid nitrogen canisters. It has nothing to do with the plague resting in a Biosafety Level 3 facility; therefore, there is no need for art history to engage with the zoonotic dimension of the disease, or come to terms with the notion of zoonotic diagram and its dynamic representation of disease transmission.

Barker's stance on Poussin's pestilence seems fair and her historicism sound, but does it mean that the painting is dead to the world in which it survived? The injunction to "suspend our contemporary conceptions of plague and human biology" could also read like a containment protocol that seeks to preserve the painting's historical content from a contaminating present that knows nothing about the early modern theories on plague etiologies. If so, the question is not about whether frightening representations of the plague caused or could cause harm, or by what biological or psychosomatic mechanisms modern medicine might seek to understand how the psychological distress induced by an image could induce death or at least make someone sick? Rather, it is about whether it is possible to solicit early modern memories of pestilence in the epidemiological present in which *The Plague of Ashod* survives, as something else than a cache of frightening images anticipating on our worst-case scenarios, or as something else than a future-perfect held in abeyance by the governance of emerging infectious diseases? These questions are warranted by the fact that early modern memories of pestilence have been weaponized before. Frightening images may not be understood anymore to infect bodies and minds in an art historical context, but stigmatizing representations and stereotypes about infectious diseases continue to cause harm.

Of course, Barker is right. Pestilence in *The Plague of Ashod* designates an affective state of affairs rather than a microbiological reality. By the same token, the plague in Poussin's painting is less an object of governance than a public spectacle with a theatrical depth. But in a way, the same could be said of the meningoencephalitis virus one (MEV-1) in Soderbergh's pandemic thriller *Contagion* (2011). MEV-1 was imagined in consultation with Ian Lipkin, a molecular biologist and, at the time, the director of the Northeast Biodefense Center, as a fictional crossover between the Hendra and Nipah viruses. Lipkin explained that "this particular virus doesn't just cause respiratory disease. It gets into the brain and results in seizures and coma and death, which made it much more exciting and interesting, because there's a lot more you can do with it than just watching people gasping for breath" (2011, 1219). This means that, keeping Woolf's remark about influenza and the novel in mind, a plot may even have the chance to develop. As viruses go, some are more camera ready than others. But the reality is, Jameson (2010, 366–368) would say, good plots are hard to get by after modernism anyway. Ultimately, pestilence may very well drive the plot to its exhaustion but until it does, the outbreak narrative remains a steady source of narrative formulas in a permissive global urban world running out plot and plot-driving motives. Because viral life doesn't need motives to spread and conquer the world, only evolutionary opportunities, it was only "natural," so to speak, for the figure of the emerging virus to join the rank of the maniac, the serial killer, and the terrorist as a new category of faceless evil and for the epidemiological thriller to emerge as a genre at the end of the twentieth century.[1]

Lipkin responded to the narrative challenge of a film devoted to an influenza-like pandemic by devising a fictional virus that could drive a good plot. When asked about his involvement in the making of *Contagion* as a scientific consultant and the reasons he did "bother inventing a virus that doesn't really exist," he answered that he "wanted to come up with a plausible explanation for why this thing became so much more pathogenic and capable of transmitting to humans." In itself Lipkin's remark is not that interesting, except that it comes from a long line of pronouncements regarding the aesthetic and moral grounds on which fictional characters are invented. In that regard, the M1V backstory is more than a testament to Soderbergh's commitment to technical accuracy. The creation of synthetic viruses is embedded in the moral fabric of contemporary microbiology. In fact, as spectators were flocking to see *Contagion* in theaters, a Dutch virologist from Erasmus University was stirring controversy in

---

[1] For a recent assessment of the metaphorical conflation between terrorism and virus see Kolb (2020).

the highest spheres of public health and biosecurity after it had been announced that he had created a highly transmissible version of avian flu (H5N1) as a proof of concept. To show that a dangerous mutation of an existing virus could exist, a dangerous version of the virus was brought into existence (Keck 2015). A new and daring take on the old notion of verisimilitude if there is any!

The dialectic between actual outbreaks and fictional epidemic events was already an object of discussion in the work of René Girard on scapegoating mechanisms and social transgression in the 1970s. Why is it that "the plague, as a literary theme, is still alive today, in a world less and less threatened by real bacterial epidemics"? This paradoxical fact, he continues:

> looks less surprising now, as we come to realize that the properly medical aspects of the plague never were essential; in themselves, they always played a minor role, serving mostly as a disguise for an even more terrible threat that no science has ever been able to conquer. The threat is still very much with us, and it would be a mistake to consider the presence of the plague in our literature as a matter of formal routine, as an example of a tradition that persists even though its object has vanished. (1974, 845)

In Girard's argument, the moment of epidemiological transition relegating epidemic infectious diseases to the past has a purifying effect on literary memories of pestilence. It reveals plague motifs to their allegorical or anthropological essence. Again, the point seems fair but infectious threats are still very much with us. In fact, the contemporary proliferation of pandemic scenarios and outbreak narratives that organize our relation to threat and fictions of unconquerable threats would be inconceivable without the shift in the discourse of public health away from the "epidemiological transition" hypothesis, which envisioned the end of the war on viruses, toward the emerging infectious disease (EID) paradigm introduced by microbiologist Stephen Morse in the late 1980s. After the eradication of smallpox in the 1970s, the World Health Organization declared a time of epidemiological transition but the prospects of a future without germs did not last long. A negative futurity showed up in virulent zoonotic forms: AIDS, Ebola, Hantavirus, SARS, zika, COVID-19, monkeypox… etc. It is showing up yet again in the form of antibiotic resistance. Does it mean that the definition of a new state of permanent viral and bacterial warfare under the EID rubric should affect negatively the value of Girard's reading of pestilence as a literary theme? The representation of an emergent infectious epidemic event often carries the same motifs as a late medieval plague parable. Scapegoating mechanisms, the rewriting of social hierarchies, the collapse of political and moral orders: none of these patterns are absent from a movie like *Contagion*. In other words, recent developments in the epidemiology of infectious disease have no impact on the value of Girard's interpretation of the plague as a literary theme because mythical elements of threat and what he calls "social plagues" remain at work in the making of contemporary outbreak narratives. Contemporary pandemic cinema may be informed by the latest development in virology, microbiology, and epidemiology but it is clear that it doesn't let go completely of retributive narrative mechanisms. The pervasiveness of the moral discourse surrounding cinema as medium of moral corruption in the 1930s returns with a vengeance in *Outbreak* (1995, dir. Wolfgang Petersen), most explicitly in the scene where the movie theater becomes a super spreading site for the deadly airborne pathogen.[2] In *Contagion*, the lethal virus thrives in the vicinity of illicit encounters and the adulterous woman ends up dying first in the most graphic manner.

On the other hand, Girard's thesis cannot simply brush off the emergence of new infectious diseases. His treatment of pestilence as literary motif posited a status quo, according to which it was unnecessary for literary and cultural theory to engage with the epidemiological world. As the idea of epidemiological transition and its promises of collective health came to pass, couldn't we say that the relation between epidemiology and literature has been reopened and is now awaiting to be reassigned? However, does it mean that epidemiologists ought to have the last word on *The Plague of Ashod*? It would be quite a pity since epidemiology has nothing interesting to say about the painting, or about painting for that matter. Putting the plague back in Poussin's painting as *Yersinia pestis* is mostly helpful as a way to come to terms with the fact that epidemiology does not account for the existence of the painting as a work of art. Here, epidemiology is not a source of explanations. It is what returns us to the puzzlement of representation—starting with the puzzling point of entry into *Contagion* (Fig. 11.1).

---

[2] For a detailed analysis of this scene see Ostherr (2005, 187–188).

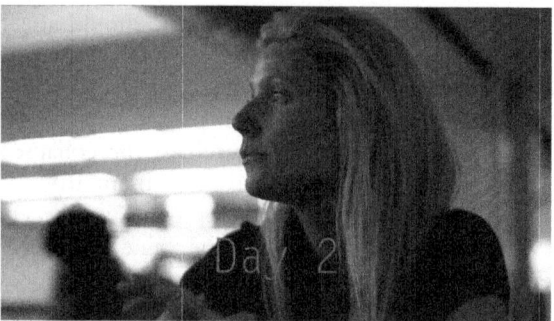

Fig. 11.1 *Contagion.* Day 2

The opening act of *Contagion* is explosive and yet easy to overlook. The first image is a non-image that consists in a blackout screen captioned by the faint verbal trail of what appears to be an airport announcement punctuated by the sound of someone coughing. Cut to the face of a woman—Beth Emhoff played by Gwyneth Paltrow—putting something in her mouth and coughing again, while "Day 2" appears in red letters at the bottom of the screen. A lot is at stake in these two delays: sound before image; Day 2 before Day 1. A key narrative element went missing, as if something did not register properly. Unless the missing link is the blank screen itself, since the airport announcement in the background is directly connected to the opening image. The dry cough, however, remains uncontained by the absence of image. It is unframed, unchecked, and more importantly unassigned to a body. It is in that sense that *Contagion*'s opening act has an explosive quality. By contrast, the close-up view of a sneeze filmed in slow motion against a dark background at 2000 frames per second is predicated on visual containment. It assigns a space and a velocity to the dispersion of droplets traveling as far as twenty-six feet. But because the image was released in JAMA (the Journal of the American Medical Association) at a time where social distancing recommendations insisted on a 6-feet separation, it also registers the meaninglessness of what is essentially a spasm as a socially significant event. And it is as such that it became one of the visuals that defined the contours of the pandemic present in March 2020 as a time of heightened anxiety over the mode of transmission of the COVID-19 virus in public spaces.

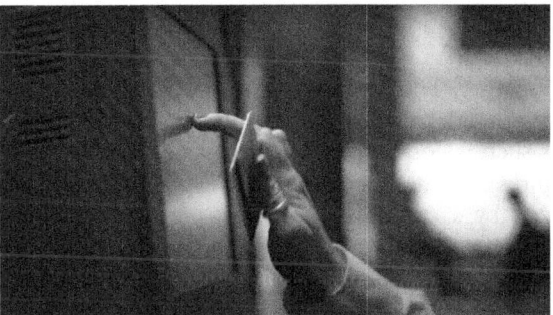

Fig. 11.2   One in a billion of unmonitored contagion events. *Contagion*

Mary Anne Doane (1980, 40) observes that "the use of the voice-off always entails a risk." It puts at risk the cinematic apparatus marrying bodies to the sounds that come from them. The opening "cough-off" in *Contagion* recasts the cinematic risk in epidemiological terms. It blurs the boundaries between the symptomatic and the narrative body, between bodies that cough and bodies that engage in conquest and conspiracy—the very stuff outbreak narratives are made of. In the darkness of the theater, before clear boundaries between the space of the movie and the space that contains movie-goers have been established by the image on the screen, the dry cough is anybody's cough, in or off-screen. The resounding void of this opening act points to the nowhere of transmission. It anticipates on the numerous shots in the rest of the movie whose narrative import will only become apparent after the fact, less invisible than unnoticeable at first as one in a billion of unmonitored contagion events already intuited by "The Horla" ("Everything around us, everything we see without looking, everything we brush past without knowing it") (Fig. 11.2).

Finger to bowl of peanuts, peanut and finger to mouth, finger to cellphone, cellphone to face, finger back to the bowl of peanuts, finger to credit card, credit card in someone's else fingers, new set of fingers to the digital registry of a bar in a busy airport. This choreography of gestures is deeply Poussinian in Barker's description of *The Plague of Ashod*: "Extending from one end to the other is a great concatenation of human bodies linked by their reaching, touching, grasping, and leaning, each creating a dangerous possibility of human-to-human contagion. Poussin draws special attention to this physical contact between individuals by designating in several cases the precise instant when that contact occurs" (Barker 2004, 665). The difference is that in *Contagion* touch is perfunctory. The body that touches is disembodied and consists mostly of fingers and an aggregate of invisible fingerprints. It rarely has a face and as such is condemned to remain unexpressive (as opposed to Poussin's figures). If the encounter between cinema and epidemiology is characterized by a compulsion "to visually represent invisible contagions in order to fix the location of the ever-elusive pathogen," as Kirsten Ostherr writes, in Poussin's depiction of a biblical pestilence, the visuality of contagion serves another purpose (Ostherr 2005, 2). When he paints touch and contagion, Poussin gives us to see tears in the fabric of a social world. When Soderbergh films disembodied touch and cough, he alludes to the deceitfulness of surfaces and empty spaces that are never as innocent or clean as they seem to be, and thus to invisible mode of transmission (Fig. 11.3).

In the age of emerging infectious diseases, the theaters of pestilence are cinematic. Epidemiology is never more at home in cinema than in instances of sudden cuts bridging distant geographies. This move is exemplified by the juxtaposition between images of an equatorial forest (standing for the exotic source of danger and impurity *over there*) and a research facility in Maryland (standing for the national body under attack *right here*) in the opening sequence of *Outbreak*. In plague paintings and other early modern theaters of pestilence, the oscillation is between effects and affects. When the Marquis de Sade described one of the ghoulish dioramas realized in wax by Gaetano Zumbo, representing the inside of "a sepulcher filled with an infinity of corpses, in each of which one can observe the different gradients of decomposition, from the corpse of the day, to the one that worms have completely devoured," the observation would be incomplete if he did not add that the impression left by the morbid tableau was so strong that senses triggered each other: "The hand unknowingly seeks to cover the nose" (Sade 1973, 152–153).

The same gesture has a very different meaning in *Contagion*. During a briefing with officials at the Minnesota Department of Public Health, Dr. Erin Mears (Kate Winslet) explains that "the average person touches their face two or three thousand times a day, [...] three to five times every waking minute. In between, we are touching doorknobs, water fountains, elevator buttons, and each other. Those things become fomites." The juxtaposition between Sade's description and Soderbergh's cinema of contagion gives a contrastive sense of how different the two theaters of

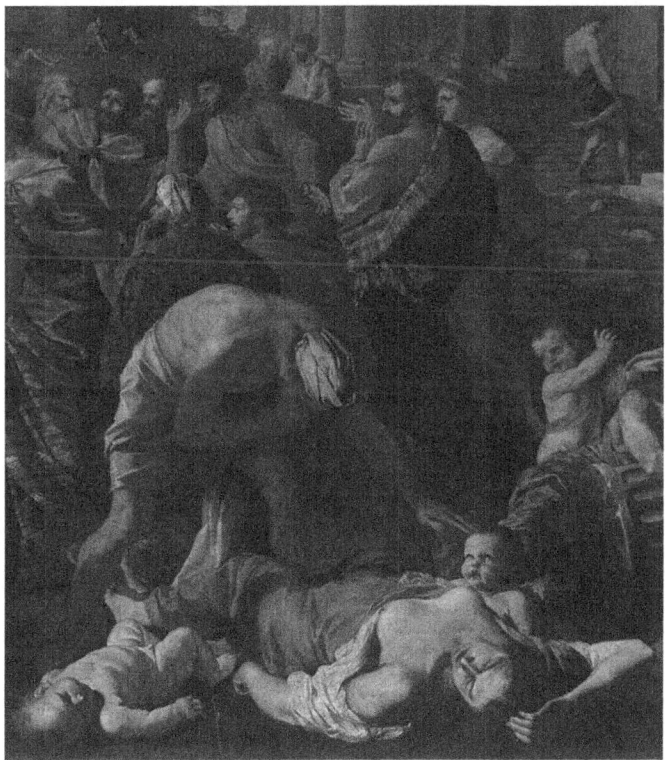

Fig. 11.3 Detail. Nicolas Poussin, *The Plague of Ashdod* (1630). Oil on canvas, 58 in. × 78 in. Louvre, Paris

pestilence are. The juxtaposition also gives us a sense of epidemiology's investment in image making. Whereas Sade dreams of a unified sensuous field, the epidemiology of emerging infectious diseases projects a unified field where contact becomes visible and actionable in the form of diagrams and network analysis (as in Fig. 11.4).

There is more to the pedagogical dimension of *Contagion* than Dr. Mears's crash course about fomites and R-naught number (R0). The movie teaches us to understand epidemiology as a defamiliarizing intuition about the world where things and bodies continuously overlap, and where the overlapping of things and bodies is more driven by habits rather than it is by motives. In linear perspective, represented objects overlap on

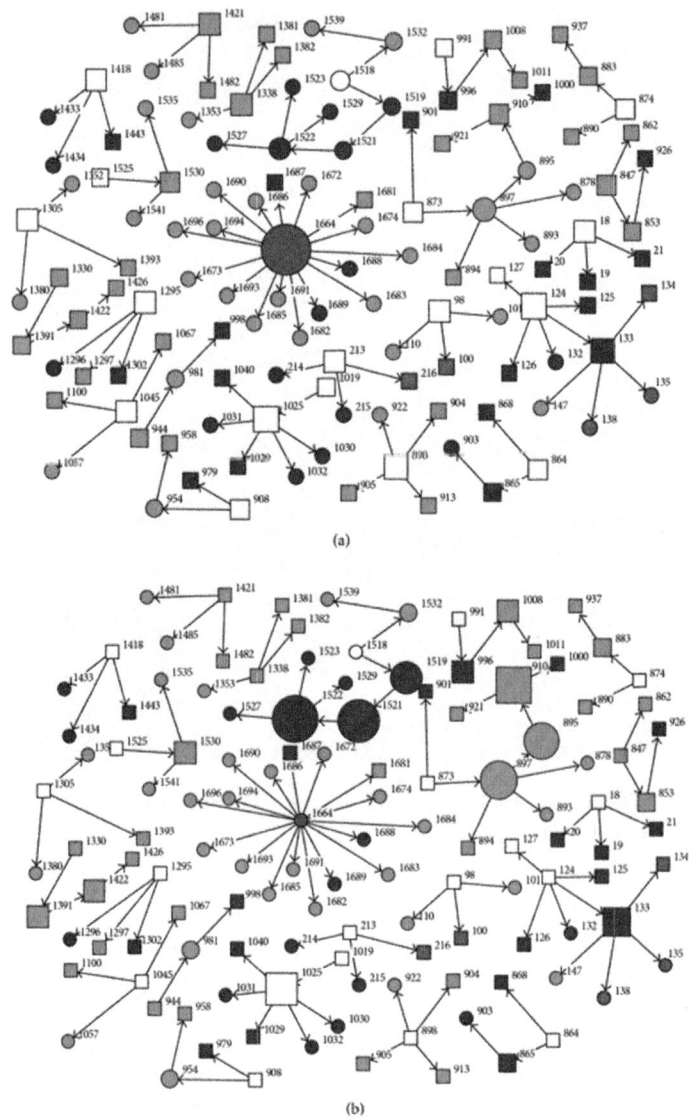

Fig. 11.4 Network contact structure for the spread of MERS-CoV infection (Oyelola A. Adegboye and Faiz Elfaki 2018)

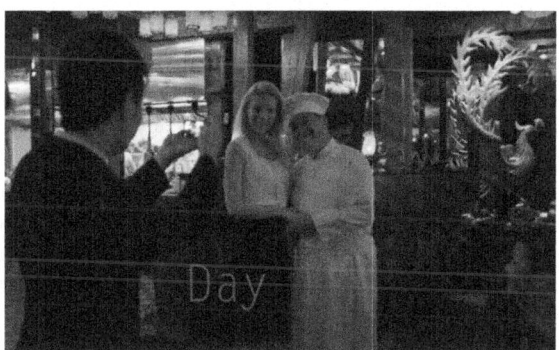

Fig. 11.5 Day 1. *Contagion*

the surface but they are understood to not touch in reality. That over-lapping is mitigated by recourse to radiating patterns that issue from a point on the horizon. In *Contagion*, epidemiology registers as an invitation to leave aside—if only for a few seconds—that visual grammar for another syntax, where contagion is the organizing principle rather than an accidental occurrence.

On "Day 4," Beth convulses and dies. By "Day 29," 26 million people will have died of the virus worldwide. The MEV-1 pandemic is eventually contained by the promise of a vaccine, which means that the series of days was after all a countdown toward the solution bringing the thriller to a close. But in a remarkable narrative move, the closing sequence of *Contagion* returns us to ground zero as a site of human animal interactions: a bulldozer takes down a palm tree and dislodges bats, one of the dislodged bats meets a pig, the pig meets its fate in the kitchen of a restaurant, where the cook greets one of his high-profile patrons, Beth Emhoff. Together, they pose for a picture on what will have been Day 1 of the global health crisis (Fig. 11.5).

After 100 minutes or so of storytelling predicated on the social and political unravelling of the world, *Contagion*'s coda brings a semblance of clarity on the origins of the pandemic crisis and a certain sense of closure, as if survivors in a post-pandemic future had finally regained a full narrative command over the unaccounted interactions (contact, contagion, contamination, transmission, mutation... etc.) that make up the epidemiological world. But Day 1 is not narrated from the perspective of a human subject. It consists in "a series of 'cuts' spliced together"

(Dixon and Jones 2014, 228). While the last image of the film exists as photograph, the scenes of contagion that led to that moment, whose status as moment is both captured by the camera and signaled by the flash, are restituted as images from nowhere. They are the equivalent of a spillover hypothesis in a zoonotic diagram (Fig. 11.6): it represents what must have happened somewhere somehow for the world to end up there, trapped in a moment of pandemic conflation. The chiasmus between the beginning and the end, between the flash and the sneeze, functions as a reminder that somewhere else another bat will meet another pig, leading to the emergence of a new mutations.

What comes first? Is it the bat, the bulldozer, the pig, the cross-contamination incident in the kitchen, or the international mobility of Beth?[3] Is it the series of incidental interactions among animals, between animals and humans, and among humans, or the hierarchical integration of these relations into the system that assign meaning to them? That is to say, where did things go wrong? Is it when the bulldozer entered the forest, when the bat dropped a chewed banana in the pig's troth, when the pig was bred, raised and killed for its meat, when the cook didn't wash his hands, when Beth traveled to Asia for work, or when she accepted to work for the mining company that owns the bulldozer that took down the palm tree? With the image of the palm tree dropping its dangerous fruit in mind, do we need to go back further in time, to remember that, for Saint Augustine, the original sin passed on with birth is the source of all contagions?[4]

The indeterminacy of *Contagion*'s opening non-image meets a different kind of indeterminacy at the end. Perhaps, the film does not bother to unbraid the strands of causality and blame because in the end, it is not up to a film to assign the difference between physical causa-tion and social causation—that is, the contact between things on the one hand, and the integration of the contact between thing into an order

---

[3] "This is day one. And it is also the beginning of the end. And no one saw it coming because Beth's mobility is presumed natural in the global order of things" (Benton 2020).

[4] On the theology of contagion see Fossier (2011). Fragments from the Augustinian tradition seem to have survived well into the twentieth century. Geddes Smith writes in *Plague on Us* (1941): "chief source of infection for mankind... is mankind itself. Most of the communicable diseases from which men suffer are kept in circulation, like original sin, by the human race." Cited in Wald (2008, 21).

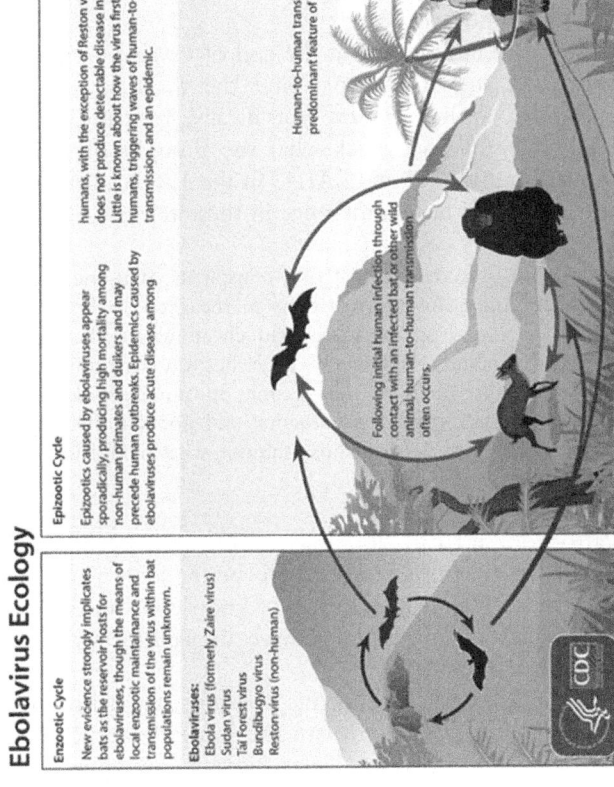

Fig. 11.6 Ebolavirus ecology. CDC infographic

that constitutes its meaning on the other.[5] But it does not mean that causation does not matter, or that unassigned differences are not without consequences. It doesn't mean either that fiction does not have something to tell us about epidemiological realities in a world where long-term patterns of rising temperatures create pathways for fungus to colonize warm-blooded creatures and provides ancient microorganisms trapped in permafrost with ecological opportunities to resurface (Sirucek 2012). If there is such a thing as epidemiological realism, it is in part because modern societies experience transmissibility and contagion both as social facts and as problems of governance.

Perhaps, this narrative indifference at the end of *Contagion* is a necessary step to break the storytelling spell and the thrill of the what-if scenario. It is akin to a shrug—more specifically, to Cindy Patton's "shrug" when asked by Eve Sedgwick what she thought of conspiracy theories circulating about the origin of AIDS in the 1980s. A nonplussed Patton reportedly explained her indifference in these terms:

> Suppose we were sure of every element of a conspiracy: that the lives of Africans and African Americans are worthless in the eyes of the United States; that gay men and drug users are held cheap where they aren't actively hated; that the military deliberately researches ways to kill noncombatants whom it sees as enemies; that people in power look calmly on the likelihood of catastrophic environmental and population changes. Supposing we were ever so sure of all those things—what would we know then that we don't already know? (2003, 123)[6]

It's not that Patton doesn't care about what virology has to say about the origins of HIV, or that origin stories are better left to mythology. Her shrug refuses to let the weaponization of knowledge and ignorance prevail over the mechanisms in place that have allowed for a population to become a target in the first place.

One thing is certain, the MV1 pandemic does not start with the non-image of Beth's cough on Day 2 but with the movie Soderbergh made about it. After all, as Ostherr explains, if there is such a thing as a cinema of contagion, it is because there are no pro-filmic images of contagion.

---

[5] On the distinction between physical and social causations see Keck (2019, 30).

[6] I borrow the image of the shrug to Anahid Nersessian's reading of the same passage in *The Calamity Form: On Poetry and Social Life* (2020, 8).

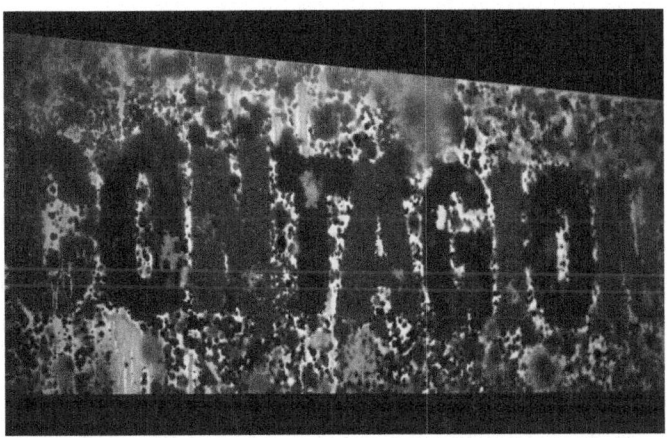

Fig. 11.7 *Contagion* billboard, 409 Queen West Toronto, 2011

Instead, we have visual and narrative proxies filling in the perceptual gaps that exist between the reality of pathogens and the realism of bodies in contact with plotlines, digital images, animated sequences, and, often-times, stigmatizing stereotypes. Or in the case of Soderbergh's pandemic thriller, the gap is filled by a sensational billboard consisting of two over-sized rectangular petri dishes coated with nutrient gel and inoculated with fungi and bacteria. Illegible at first, the word "CONTAGION" appeared in hues of pale green and vivid coral red as the cultures devel-oped over the course of the week preceding the release of the movie in Toronto (Fig. 11.7). Again, what comes first? Is it the indexicality of the growth that makes up the microbial billboard, or the artificiality of the symbolic system that subtends the use and spelling of "contagion"—the word and the idea? Is it the MV1 pandemic or the movie Soderbergh made about it? Because the MV1 pandemic is confined to the screen, the question doesn't really make sense. All it does is leave us in the dark with the disembodied cough that marks the spot where events and their recounting part ways. Until they meet again.

* * *

Confinement Notes (June 2020): *Contagion* is trending on Netflix. Even though I have already watched the movie more times I care to count, I can't help it. This time, however, it is different. The mind wanders somewhere else looking for a sense of reassurance, like the future in "This too shall pass" seen on a sticker. I'm thinking about the movie that one day will be made about life in the COVID present.[7] But isn't this movie already in production? It is composed of an indefinite number of online sessions of various length mimicking real-life interactions, some recorded, some not, and others recorded, or not recorded by mistake. It has been in the making since the beginning of the confinement period and even predates it. It tells the story of people trying to catch up, reach out, get things done, teach, learn, argue, and tear up at a distance. The public will say the movie lacks plot. It is essentially conversational, a rehearsal of familiar scripts in absentia. The content is ordinary. It improvised ordinariness in extraordinary times. Of course, it is not really a movie. And yet, we already remember our favorite scenes and the most unfortunate moments. Or else, it is a movie that only survives in fragmented memories distributed across a group of friends, colleagues, and family members, learning on-screen that reality is not a given but the shaky result of storytelling habits at the mercy of a coughing spell.

---

[7] Several commentators have equated the repetitiveness of life in the COVID present reference to the narrative loop of *Groundhog Day* (1993). See Altschuler (2021), "After the Outbreak. Narrative, Infrastructure, and Pandemic Time," 136–137.

CHAPTER 12

Scenes of Immunization (*Driftwood* 1947)

Abstract Compared to *Contagion*, *Driftwood* (1947), directed by Allan Dwan, is a quaint zoonotic fable, whose version of epidemiological realism explores the modalities of a shared living situation on the American frontier. Everybody has a lesson in cohabitation to learn in the fictional small town of Panbucket, Nevada. The ticks that transmit spotted fever do not learn. Because they bite and infect regardless of class distinctions, class distinction has to be reinvented in the guise of immunization.

Keywords *Driftwood* (film) · Immunization · Jeremiad · Rocky Mountain spotted fever · Ticks · Zoonosis

Compared to *Contagion*, Hollywood oldie, *Driftwood* (1947), directed by the prolific Allan Dwan, is much less ambitious in its narrative program. It is a quaint zoonotic fable, whose version of epidemiological realism explores the modalities of a shared living situation with the ticks that transmit Rocky Mountains spotted fever in the American West. Everybody has a lesson in cohabitation to learn in the small town of Panbucket, Nevada. Steve Webster, or Doc Steve—the local doctor conducting research on infected ticks—needs to settle down and learn his way to financial independence. Sue, his devoted love interest, learns what it takes to become someone's wife. An old bickering couple, Murph and Mathilda, whose relationship has not been formalized yet, gives another wobbling go at courtship with a brash no-nonsense attitude. Wide-eyed orphan Jenny learns the ways of a world that is not governed by the Scriptures but by external markers of class—and possibly of race, although the movie remains completely silent on the subject.

At first, Jenny's bible-quoting righteousness and raggedy clothes make her stand out, but she learns fast, starts to blend in, gets a bath, new clothes, and a cream soda. Along the way she picks up new words and notions:

> Jenny—If you're the doctor, you have to go about the land and heal with the laying on of your hands.
> Doc Steve—Well, it's not that simple. See our laying on of hands is different. Today we call it "therapeutics."
> Jenny—Therap, thera...
> Doc Steve—peutics
> Jenny—peutics?
> Doc Steve—Hmm. Or "Prophylaxis"
> Jenny—Pro-fuh...
> Doc Steve—...phylaxis
> Jenny—prophylaxis
> Doc Steve—That's right. And we use chemicals and serums and vaccines. See, that's the miracle that keep people from having disease. Reminds me, I better vaccinate you right away.

But "right away" never comes. Panbucket's scheming mayor barges in looking for the dog that allegedly attacked his son when he threatened Jenny. He makes a scene and makes a mess on the porch where ticks are kept in stacked-up glass containers. The distracted doctor leaves the girl unvaccinated and vulnerable.

Immunization does not eradicate ticks. It makes their existence compatible with that of the settlers by minimizing the disruption they might cause. Unlike Jenny, the ticks that transmit spotted fever do not learn. Because at Mathilda's dismay, they bite and infect regardless of class distinctions, class distinction has to be reinvented in the guise of immunization. Immunization impresses the social difference that Sunday dresses and hair ribbons fail to achieve. Like a manicured appearance, it is a distinction that can be learned. The town's good people learn the virtue of immunization from the cautionary tale of unvaccinated young Clem Perkins succumbing to spotted fever.[1] Ticks may not be socially discerning but at the same time, the plotline suggests that people living on the margins are more likely to be infected with less favorable outcomes. The Perkins family is marked by poverty. They live outside town in a more modest home that the camera dare not enter. It means that Jenny is the next logical victim: she too is unvaccinated and she too comes from the social fringes. Fortunately, she is also far enough along in the civilization process initiated by Doc Steve to be rescued.

Her salvation comes in extremis in the form of a serum extracted from the stray dog *ex machina* that she found at the beginning of the movie. A convoluted plot twist reveals that the border collie is in fact a retired lab animal that not only survived a plane crash but whose blood happens to contain the very antibodies Jenny needs to fight the fever. She lives through the night and wakes up into a world where everything around her neatly falls into place, or rather units—husband, wife, child, and housedog—but also as science and faith. For in the end, Jenny is saved by the serum as much as she is healed by the pastor's prayers. His sententious words of wisdom—"If a thing can be done science and skill can do it. If a thing cannot be done only faith can do it"—strike the ultimate worlding deal. It's tenuously rhetorical at best but it will have to do for now—if only for the sake of bringing the fable to a close. But not for long in the greater scheme of things.[2]

It is easy to forget that *Driftwood* is a tale of two settlements: bustling Panbucket, where most of the action takes place, and desolate Bullfrog Springs, which was "once the queen of the gold rush days." Don't be fooled by the tumbleweeds and the arid landscape, the opening shot of *Driftwood* belongs to the ruined world painted by Poussin in *The Plague of Ashod*. Even the plane crash showering the earth with fire is evocative of the ancient belief in the meteoric dimension of pestilence. A tired preacher

---

[1] See Conis (2015, 3): "Before the 1960's [...] vaccination in the United States was typically an individual, local, and reactive affairs. Parents vaccinated children to protect them from feared diseases."

[2] Rosenberg gives 1945 as a breaking point in the US, after which the ideal of compatibility between scientific innovation and spiritual values of justice and charity will have to make way for a new political reality and a new generation of epidemiological fables (1973, 233). See also Cronon (2011, x): "Whereas an earlier era had habitually looked to science and technology for solutions to social and environmental problems, by the 1960s these agents of 'progress' [...] seemed as often as not to cause those problems."

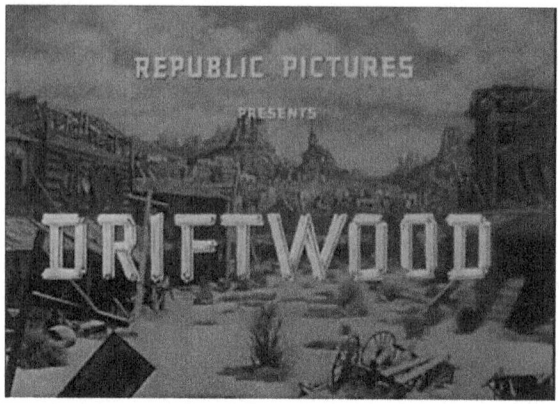

Fig. 12.1   Opening credits. *Driftwood*

in the American wilderness, Reverend Hollingsworth reads from Jeremiah 1 verse 6 ("Then said I, Ah, Lord God! behold, I cannot speak: for I am a child.") before collapsing in front of her great-granddaughter, Jenny, who has no choice but to flee Bullfrog Springs (Fig. 12.1).

No explanation is provided regarding what led a settlement to prosper and the other to collapse but let's assume for the sake of argument that spotted fever is to be blamed. In Panbucket, the disease is understood to be endemic. It threatens the integrity of the settlement, forcing its population to reconvene and to immunize their offspring. In the jeremiad tradition, sickness is providential.[3] It strikes a community and has to be endured as a divine trial. Pestilence is a litmus test around which to reorganize one's sense of belonging, or election, or belonging through election. There is no room for inoculation in this scenario, not even as an opt-in procedure. Life in common (and under God) is contagious by design. It is shaped by exposure, death, and remission. Sickness and health are not a matter of personal choice or politics. In Bullfrog Springs, spotted fever was an object of reckoning. In Panbucket, it has become an object of governance.

---

[3] On the epidemiological underpinnings of the jeremiad tradition in colonial New England see Silva (2011).

CHAPTER 13

The Rabid Wolf and the Sovereign (Bauhin 1591; Lafontaine 1668)

Abstract The prospects of a future without germs that gained traction in the 1970s did not last long. A negative futurity showed up in virulent zoonotic forms. It is showing up yet again in the form of antibiotic resistance. The Emerging Infectious Disease (EID) paradigm creates an opening insofar as it subsumes, in the words of Frédéric Keck and Christos Lynteris, "all human-animal coexistence [...] under the sign of the 'coming plague', every human-animal interaction becomes a potential pandemic ground zero"—even, and against all odds, or so I argue in Vignette 13, the human–animal interactions described in the chronicle of a rabies outbreak that occurred in 1590 on the border between France and Germany.

Keywords Bauhin · Jean · Drought · Ecology · Lafontaine, Jean de · Preventive measures · Rabies · Wolves · Zoonosis

This vignette too revolves around a zoonotic event straddling secular and scriptural dispensations. Jean Bauhin's *Histoire Notable de la Rage des Loups* is the chronicle of a local rabies outbreak that occurred in 1590 in Eastern France near Montbéliard. A situation has developed consisting in a series of incidents: a wolf is sighted near x where it attacks α and then

© The Author(s), under exclusive license to Springer Nature
Switzerland AG 2024
V. Bruyere, *Epidemiological Realism*, Palgrave Studies in Literature,
Science and Medicine,
https://doi.org/10.1007/978-3-031-68517-0_13

goes to z where it attacks β, and so on and so forth. The chronological gridding of the incursions is precise and yet muddied by the recent transition from Julian to Gregorian calendar ("June, the 25th according to the old calendar, and July the 5th according to the new, a Thursday morning at 9 o'clock in the seignory of Belfort, in a village called Bourongne…" [Bauhin 1591, 7–8]). Each attack is followed by a description of the wounds inflicted by the animal, the period of incubation before the development of neurological symptoms characteristics of the disease such as hydrophobia, and finally the conditions in which the victim died.

The first series of attacks ends when a red she-wolf is killed after a 24-hour rampage that makes twelve victims and claims nine lives at the time of the retelling—the period of incubation before the apparitions of neurological symptoms can be quite long, so it might not have been over by the time of the *Histoire*'s publication in 1591. It is followed by a second rampage that is geographically adjacent and may or may not be related to the first one, with more than forty sightings and/or attacks resulting in at least five deaths. Five animals are killed but it is not clear how many wolves are involved in the second string of attacks.

After the retelling of the two outbreaks, Bauhin offers a compendium of remedies gleaned in classical and contemporary treaties but, in a sense, the retelling itself is already a remedy. It mends at a narrative level what the lupine incursions have unstitched at a territorial level. With this account, Bauhin presents the sovereign and the local dignitaries to which the *Histoire* is dedicated with the verbal map of a territory under attack, which at a basic level makes the outbreak a political event. However, what is being redrawn by Bauhin's mapping gesture are less the outer-contours of a territory than species boundaries, understood as a theologico-political construct rather than as a biological fact. For what appears to be under attack in Montbéliard and Belfort is the dominion of men over the natural kingdom:

> May God give to the rulers [*les grands*] the will, the courage, the strength, assistance and dexterity to extirpate the wolves and prevent them from doing wrong, according to the power they received from God, Genesis 1, when he commands that Man would rule over the fishes of the sea, and the birds of the sky, and the beasts, and over the entire earth, and over all the reptiles that crawl on the earth. (1591, 41)

This connection between parts and whole, between the vernacular and the scriptural intuited by Bauhin's narrative accounts for the far-reaching significance of the outbreak no matter how confined or contained the series of incidents is. Because the crisis he recounts in his *Histoire* concerns the very fabric of the world in which the rabid incursions occurred, I'm almost tempted to say that there is something "pandemic" about an otherwise eminently local epidemic event.

In epidemiology, the conjectural moment where a pathogen jumps from its animal reservoir to a human population—or put differently, the point of entry of animal life and death into the realm of human affairs and mastery over Nature—is called a spillover. A spillover event is a narrative placeholder that allows for a series of incidents to register *après coup* as a zoonotic event. In lieu of a spillover event, Bauhin gives us a long list of biblical admonitions involving animal attacks motivated by divine wrath and revenge and comes to the following conclusion: "Let's take at heart these threats that God offers through his Holy Scriptures, and now let's take note of what began in these quarters in the year 1590 (the heat and drought having been most severe, and for many years unseen to such a degree in these lands)" (1591, 7). The mention of a dry year could be an ecological element of explanation. It could point in the direction of a triggering disturbance, but in Bauhin's *Histoire,* it only functions as a chronicling element. The 1590 outbreak comes from nowhere. Or rather, it comes from a place—the Scriptures—that is not assignable in the vernacular register that accounts for it. The disturbed humanimal relations in Montbéliard and the humanimal status in Genesis 1 belong to different realms brought together to represent the rabid incursions as something else than a series of incidents.

If the references to the Scriptures and the prescriptions on how to "treat" rabies gathered by Bauhin situate the local rabies outbreak in relation to a long-term memory of pestilence, the narrative retelling situates the attacks in a pastoral landscape of orchards, farms, and meadows, where children pick up cherries, girls gather simples, and women tend farm animals. These vignettes form the social context in which the rabies outbreak occurs and the incidents aggregate. What's realist in Bauhin's prose hinges on a tacit commitment to representing human affairs as the narrative backdrop of epidemic circumstances. What's epidemiological in his realism hinges on the overlapping between the narrative recording of homely realia and the quasi-forensic logic behind their incidental representation in the margins of the rabid incursions.

In the last two pages of the chronicle, the pastoral disruption is met with a concerted cynegetic movement of retaliation.[1] Bauhin repositions the outbreak in the perspective of a collective mobilization citing Jean de Clamorgan's treaty on the art of wolf hunting, in which the author instructs to "gather people in the vicinity or close to the woods or groves, where wolves dwell and retreat, and assign to members of each parish positions and spots to occupy." Clamorgan continues: "The parishioners will thus march in good order, each led by one of the troop leaders to make sure they keep rank and walk across the woods until they reach the place where the nets and webs are installed." It takes a village to rid woods and groves from its wolf population (Fig. 13.1).

The last remedy offered in Bauhin's *Histoire* by way of Clamorgan's hunting treaty does not target rabies's symptoms but its animal reservoir and the possibility of episodic recurrences. Because the vernacular origins of the rabies outbreak remain unknown, it may happen again and again. This last preemptive move shifts ever so slightly the theologico-political identity of the rabies outbreak under the sign of Genesis 1, toward matters of ecopolitics where, in the words of Keck and Lynteris (2018): "all human-animal coexistence [...] under the sign of the 'coming plague', every human-animal interaction becomes a potential pandemic ground zero"—even the human–animal interactions described in the chronicle of a rabies outbreak that occurred at the end of sixteenth century on the border between France and Germany.

The modernity of Bauhin's account is perhaps more explicitly legible in his outright dismissal of the werewolf hypothesis: the attacks are perpetrated by *Lupus canis* not by demonic men. Bauhin's wolves bite and infect domesticated animals and their humans. They are not fabulous, unlike their counterpart in Jean de Lafontaine first book of *Fables* (1668). As the story goes, a lamb drinks into a stream that does not divide anything yet. A wolf interrupts the scene to claim rights over the water by way of an accusation: "Who makes you so bold as to disturb my beverage? / Says this animal full of rage" (cited in Marin 1989, 74). Of course, Lafontaine's wolf is not exactly rabid but rather "full of rage."

In French, *rage* is both a disease and a passion. In 1690, Antoine Furetière defines *rage* as a "disease that ravishes reason and excites fury," adding: "Rage is also used in the language of moral, figuratively, to

[1] On the biblical genealogy and the biopolitical import of the opposition between hunting power and pastoral power see Lynteris (2020, 111).

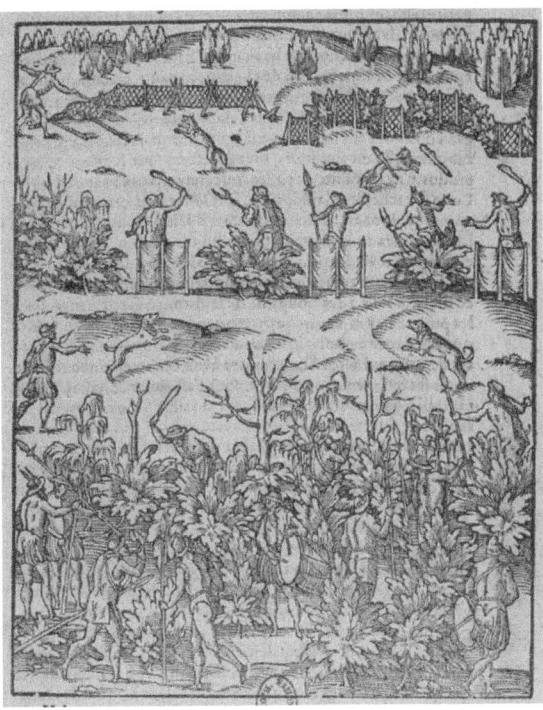

Fig. 13.1 Jean de Clamorgan. *La chasse du loup, nécessaire à la maison rustique* (1574). Chap. 20

describe unbridled passions." The semantic range of the term opens up swapping possibilities between human and animal bodies—Furetière again: "One calls enraged dog a wicked man, who seeks to do harm to others and commits vicious acts." It is in that sense that there is something strangely fabulous about zoonoses—fabulous as in the realm of fables, where fully anthropomorphized animals exchange words and play the human comedy, as well as in the realm of co-evolutionary cautionary tales teaching us that "the animal is […] part of a dynamic biological world *with which our bodies continuously swap properties*" (Braun 2008, 257). If fabulous animals are vectors of political imagination then what would it mean for fables to be vectors of zoonotic imagination?

The semantic range of "rage" comes into play with the semantic range of the word "reason" in the opening statement of Lafontaine's fable: "The reason [*raison*] of the strongest is always the best." The strongest is right (*il a raison*). The strongest prevails (*il a raison de*) (Derrida 2009, 280). It is pointless to reason with the wolf because he is in his right in the realm of the fable and will prevail. It is also pointless because he is full of rage and therefore deprived of reason. The lamb tries his best, conceding to his enraged opponent his territorial claims, while quietly claiming for himself mastery over language in a rejoinder that takes over the fable:

> Sire, replies the lamb, would that Your Majesty
> Might refrain from anger;
> Instead let Him consider that I drink
> From the Stream
> At more than twenty feet below His Majesty.
> As a consequence, I can in no way
> Disturb His drink. (Cited in Marin 1989, 76)

For a brief moment, the lamb has the upper verbal hand but it is only until the wolf manages to put his rage into words: "For you and yours hardly spare me/You, your shepherds, and your dogs" (cited in Marin 1989, 81). It appears in these lines that Lafontaine's wolf is full of rage against the agro-pastoralist machine with which he and his kind are at war. Because the wolf singles out the eloquent lamb but targets its mode of existence, his fabled rage could be interpreted as giving voice to matters of ecopolitical concern: the presence of the lamb by the stream may be a sign of pasture expansion and the conflict over access to water a sign of pressure put on shared resources.[2]

For reasons that may be obvious to veterinarians—because he killed and ate his prey—Lafontaine's fabulous wolf is not rabid but rabies looms on the horizon of the fable. The pressure it puts on the access to sources

---

[2] The incidence of rabies in twenty-first-century Madagascar is also a matter of ecopolitical disturbance because the disruption of natural habitats and the displacement of wildlife linked to large mining operations in the rain forest have created conditions in which spillover events are more likely to occur. During her fieldwork in the Moramanga District, anthropologist Genese Sodikoff (2016) discovered that these ecopolitical disturbances have found a fabulous expression in the conjectural existence of a creature believed by many on the island to be the vector of rabies infections, the *kelibetratra*, or "little big chest," a wild species of dog that no one has ever observed directly, only heard howling in the night, and by extension, only heard off.

Fig. 13.2 "The sheep of the future." Clockwise: followed by satellite, muzzle-mask, removable spine, compulsory cellphone (tracking, vaccine monitoring, travel license, social media credit score, digital money), compulsory vaccine, social distancing sensor, gender abolition, Implant, Soma (the fictional happy pill from Huxley's *Brave New World*)

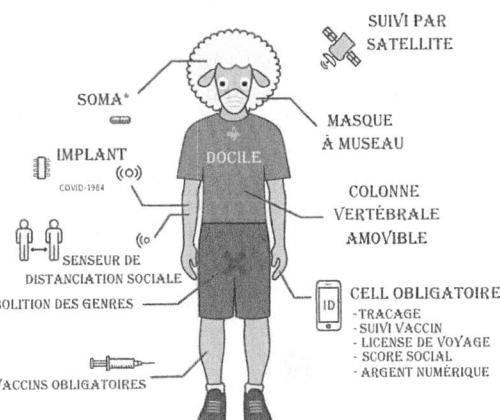

of water lines up with etiological hypotheses about rabies incidence. A 2012 report citing Dr. Charles Rupprecht, chief of the rabies program at the CDC, "noted that [...] in the bone-dry central United States, where animals are forced to congregate at fewer and fewer available water sources, the uptick in rabid wildlife is even more pronounced" (Murphy and Wasik 2012). Furetière's dictionary also mentions that "Dogs are subject to becoming rabid during heat waves [*canicule*: literally dog-days] when they lack water." Lafontaine doesn't say anything about it but in my mind "the Wolf and the Lamb" is set on a scorching summer day and the pasture is no longer green.

Lafontaine's lamb is lost to the rage of a lone wolf but the agro-pastoralist system with which it was identified did endure and evolve so that one day, a lamb would grow up to become in the pandemic present of the COVID-19 crisis, "the sheep of the future": a fabled anthropo-morphic creature born from a sense of discontent with public health policy and governance, half-human, half-sheep, identified by the pros-thetic attributes of its innate compliance to an invisible entity (Fig. 13.2). Unlike its meek ancestor, the sheep of the future has nothing left to fear—the wolf population is either under control, reintroduced in moni-tored sanctuaries, or simply extinct—but the Orwellian/Huxleyan regime to which it owes its placid existence. It is fully medicated, vaccinated, geolocated, masked, spineless, and neutered by gender theory. Given the underlying theme, one would have almost expected for the sheep of the future to be a clone, or else subject to reproductive cloning in tribute to its distinguished counterpart Dolly (Franklin 2007). But it is also obvious that the visual fable of "The sheep of the future" was not conceived to achieve analytical coherence, only to magnetize frustration.

CHAPTER 14

Scenes of Awkwardness (*Little Joe* 2019)

Abstract This vignette engages with Benjamin Bratton's idea that the collective intelligence of epidemiological realism is achieved through sensing rather than feeling, sensing being another word for testing, and testing another way for all bodies to be seen and counted. Indeed, who cares about deeply felt forms of togetherness when a 50-milliliter sample of wastewater can be made to represent that togetherness? The fraught relation between sensing and feeling is at the core of Jessica Hausner's 2019 movie *Little Joe*, an awkward bioethical fable that doesn't care to deliver on its bioethical premises.

Keywords Epidemiology · Friction · Invasive species · *Little Joe* (film) · Sensing · Testing

"We live in an epidemiological reality" is a political statement simply by virtue of the collective representation it posits, perhaps not carefully enough. For Claire Colebrook (2020) is right: "Using the word "we" these days is not smart." But the thing is, these days, political statements are not smart; they are a matter of feeling orchestrated by representations that are affirming or rub you the wrong way—which is what epidemiological views of society tend to do; the COVID-19 pandemic

© The Author(s), under exclusive license to Springer Nature
Switzerland AG 2024
V. Bruyere, *Epidemiological Realism*, Palgrave Studies in Literature,
Science and Medicine,
https://doi.org/10.1007/978-3-031-68517-0_14

made that painfully clear. In *The Revenge of the Real*, Bratton calls for a strong version of epidemiological realism to rise above that affective state of affairs. It is his contention that collective intelligence of the world will be achieved through *sensing* rather than *feeling*—sensing being another word for testing, and testing another way for all bodies to be seen and counted. Pandemic deniers, antivaxxers, anti-maskers, technophobic metaphysicists, conspiracy theorists, and other magical thinkers can wish away the world in which they live all they want, the real will take its revenge and put an end to all the nonsense because feeling a certain way toward the world will only be met with indifference by the world and by numbers. Besides, who cares about deeply felt forms of togetherness when a 50-milliliter sample of wastewater can be made to represent that togetherness?

The distinction between feeling and sensing is seductive because of its ability to cut through the chaotic proliferation of affective responses to a situation of crisis. And so is the revenge narrative because of its ability to tap into a well-worn trope that both fits frustration like a glove and renews with a punitive and admonitory rhetoric of pestilence. That said, an epidemiological view of society may have (an admonitory version of) reality on its side but it remains a matter of (statistical) representation (informing political decision and) eliciting (strong) feelings, even as it seeks to take feelings out of the political. In other words, it may very well be that epidemiological concepts have seeped into the fabric of social life and contributed to redraw the contours of ordinariness; but not without creating a certain amount of friction between forms of collective intelligence and between modes of taking the world in that do not see the world eye to eye.

Friction between sensing and feeling is another reason why there is such a thing as epidemiological realism. In this vignette, I consider the fraught relation between sensing and feeling as mediated through the strange case of *Little Joe* (Jessica Hausner 2019) and its fantasy of a frictionless world. Alice Woodard designed Little Joe, a flowering houseplant, to be loved and named it after her teenager son, Joe. When properly cared for, Little Joe appears to bring people together by releasing the mother-hormones in its scent. United by a feeling to spread good feelings, Little Joe's converts don't even need a statement to belong. All they need is a whiff and they will do whatever it takes to protect the plant and spread a feeling. They operate with a clear sense of who is in and who is not.

Bella, one of Alice's coworkers, plays the worried outcast. She worries that Little Joe's pollen might be neurotoxic and that the plant is harnessing its neurotoxicity to compensate for its inability to reproduce by other means. She also worries because her beloved dog Bello has been exposed and had to be put down after he started to behave erratically. Her concerns soon become a source of collective annoyance and mean-spirited gossip about her mental health history. So, to elude scrutiny and the unwanted attention, Bella decides to play along. She appears to have come to her senses. She says she's back on her meds. She pretends to be fine until she can't take it anymore. After finding Bello's toy in the greenhouse—a red toy, spherical and spiked, which bears an uncanny resemblance with the flower, Bella has a meltdown in the cafeteria. Alice is starting to worry too. Not only the evidence of Little Joe's neurotoxicity is mounting but she may also be responsible for what's happening because she knowingly used an unapproved transfection method to engineer the plant. When she finally voices her concerns to her supervisor and confessed her breach of protocol, Alice appeals twice to the certainty that thorough genetic tests will bring. And twice her nonplussed supervisor appeals rhetorically to questions that are not meant to be answered: "Who can prove the genuineness of feelings? Moreover, who cares?" The exchange pits sensing against feeling to no avail.

Still, something bad is happening. It is plainly palpable in the bitter-sweet stridency of the soundtrack composed by Teiji Ito (1935–1986), with its unorthodox mix of dog barking sounds, arabesques of flute inspired by the garaku tradition, and percussive shrieks. And less so in the saturation of warm colors and the understatement of starched pastels, in the oppressive neatness of glazed surfaces and the rehearsed gestures of bodies that expertly manipulate lab instruments but rarely touch each other. The spectator is on high alert but the distress signals are not specific enough to locate the source of the problem with certainty. Thus, Hausner's film leaves us stranded between competing versions of the world: one in which Bella jumped or fell off a railing after an emotional outburst at work, and the one in which she was pushed; one in which the scent of Alice's plant has appeasing virtues and one in which it is dangerously intoxicating. In other words, is Little Joe invasive because people are emotionally deprived, consumed by their professional life, and yet left unfulfilled by its empty promises? Is Alice having problems with her son because she spends too much time at work, or is she spending too much time at work because she is having trouble coming to terms with her son's attitude toward her? Is Joe growing up, seeking more independence from his mother and inviting girls over, or is Little Joe is infecting him and absorbing his emotional energy? Is Alice's male coworker just being flirtatious, or is it a case of harassment in the workplace?

Little Joe has the allure of a cautionary tale about what happens when the biotech industry is left unchecked but fails to deliver the lesson the genre implicitly promises, if it is indeed what the depiction of speculative technology gone wrong on screen is supposed to lead to, at least by convention. The plant's invasive potential is planetary but the world it will end up contaminating is only as vast as the need to soften interpersonal relations is felt. It is as if it knew that, as Berlant puts it, the problem of the world is less alienation than the inconvenience of other people (2021, 27). Given rather dystopian premises, the ending is happy enough. Bella is in a coma. Alice has been forcefully exposed to Little Joe's pollen but appears to be in denial. The precautionary tests about Little Joe's infectious potential came back negative. Tampering may have occurred but it doesn't seem to have crossed her mind. Joe moves in with his father, relieving Alice from the guilt she felt for loving her career more than her son.

Moving away from the promise of closure built in the generic expectation associated with the outbreak narrative (as Altschuler encouraged us to do, to focus instead on infrastructures and systemic fault lines) puts epidemiological realism in an awkward position. But Hausner embraces awkwardness—that is, friction at a distance—by skirting physical and verbal confrontations and stiffening interpersonal interactions into postures. It doesn't mean *Little Joe* is entirely frictionless, quite the contrary, only that the camera work is very intentional when it comes to not registering frictions—as if frictionlessness was the solution. There is no room for the commonality of fomites in that version of epidemiological realism. Also, if the mixed reception of *Little Joe* is any indication, there are aspects of its muted horror that did rub the audience the wrong way. It is precisely in that way, that the film too is part of the sensing layer that allows the epidemiological society to represent itself, even if the terms of its representation are obviously not the same than the one that allows a wastewater sample to represent a community.

CHAPTER 15

Epilogue: The Sentinel Effect

Abstract What intermediary position can literary and cultural studies claim in an economy of knowledge driven by preparedness and predictive models? In the concluding vignette, I propose to reframe the critical gesture through the concept of sentinel introduced by Frédéric Keck as a training in attentiveness tending to the agency of elusive patterns in a state of incipiency.

Keywords Biopresent · Close reading · Epidemiology · Genre of the present · Hall, Stuart · HIV-AIDS · Sentinels

Bratton explains that "the sensing layer is made up of many different kinds of technologies, different kinds of encounters. Some of them may be quite intimate, some quite visceral, some quite distantiated, some non-tactile, some immediate, some highly mediated" (2021, 42–43). In the age of emerging infectious disease, the sensing layer also includes a range of sentinel entities—some feeling, some unfeeling: unvaccinated poultry, dendritic cells, birdwatchers, microbiologists, a territory situated at a key migratory junction, health officers and officials authorizing the culling of potentially dangerous animals, a subway railing, and a wastewater sample awaiting a panel test. According to Keck, sentinels occupy "a structural

© The Author(s), under exclusive license to Springer Nature
Switzerland AG 2024
V. Bruyere, *Epidemiological Realism*, Palgrave Studies in Literature,
Science and Medicine,
https://doi.org/10.1007/978-3-031-68517-0_15

position on a border where events occur" but they also occupy a "complex field of metaphors and practices" (2014, 51). There is an aesthetic dimension to them. For signaling, he explains, is not just about true and false alerts but also about signals that allure, dazzle, and obfuscate (see Keck 2020). The speculative existence of narrative and visual sentinels I have entertained throughout the vignettes do not warn experts against emerging diseases or outbreaks. They alert humanistic inquiry to a frightening range of possibilities and plotlines where the representation of human events is but the narrative backdrop of viral life. They bring us back to the question of how the humanities catch up with what's going on in a blatantly epidemiological world. If having something to contribute to the study of zoonoses means joining a surveillance network and engaging in statistical modeling, we are still left wondering what kind of contribution the epidemiological view of society can expect from an expertise in storytelling, narrative forms, and belatedness in an economy of knowledge driven by preparedness and predictive models.

More pointedly, in 1990, in the midst of another crisis of pandemic proportions, Stuart Hall wondered out loud: "What is the point of the study of representations, if there is no response to the question of what you say to someone who wants to know if they should take a drug and if that means they'll die two days later or a few months earlier?" (1992, 284). That humanistic inquiry would appear ill-equipped to deal in pragmatic terms with the clinical challenges of a public health emergency should not come as a surprise. Never mind that pressing pharmaceutical questions will not find answers in the study of representations; in the Kantian tradition, invoked by Erwin Panofsky forty years earlier, humanistic inquiry is essentially interested in the past. Its natural habitat is the historical record. If it is interested in the past, it is also because of its interest in reality; and the present, Panofsky explains, lacks reality. A moment ago, it was not and very soon it will be no more (1955, 23). Humanistic inquiry operates is suspended time, after the facts, in hindsight.

In the grim picture Roger Cooter paints in *Writing History in the Age of Biomedicine*, the biopresent is where historiography comes to die. He writes: "Since sociologists of science and the new neurobiological reductionists of history can presumably write all the history that is needed for contemporary culture, why bother with funding professional historians at all" (2013, 36). In this scenario, the end of history does not correspond to the end of the world but to the demise of an academic discipline that historicism had put in charge of redacting stories and assigning narrative contours to a moment in time. *Epidemiological Realism* tells a different story in which epidemiology is always more than a self-contained domain of expertise and a theater of operations—statistical or otherwise. It is also what Berlant calls a genre of the present.[1]

The meditative break, the burn-out retreat, the situation comedy, the blog entry, the twitter thread, the op-ed piece, the reboot, the remake, the spinoff, the curated soundtrack, the to-do list, and even scented candles are genres of the present tasked to assign contours to the meantime—or any stretch of time for that matter—in a more or less self-reflexive and more or less improvisational manner. Genres of the present seek answers to questions of positionality and accountability that arise in a moment of crisis (how long before the future kicks in? How soon can we talk in the past tense? Are we still in the midst of an unfolding pandemic? What is the point of the study of representations in a time of plague? Who is the "we" in "whether we want it or not, we live in an epidemiological reality?" What does it mean to want that world we are stuck in rather than to disavow its claim on us?). They offer for debate a sense of feeling historical that is not organized around dates and dating but dilation as an emotional (rather than physiological) state in which conventional temporal markers are currently unavailable and temporary rituals of telling time have to be put in place not knowing whether they will become a permanent fixture, along with new modalities of keeping track, staying in touch, venting, or retreating when necessary. Hence the presence of the scented candle on the list: if historically, marked candle have been used to tell time (and give light), a scented candle functions like an atmospheric point of anchor; it's not the Fall until the cloying smell of pumpkin spice fills the air.

German historian of ideas Reinhart Koselleck explained that the concept of historical time emerged in the post-reformation period as a response to the perceived volatility of a present "in which the determinations of experience are increasingly removed from experience itself" (2004, 4). History in that sense is a form of modeling and, as a model, a historical argument is a more or less powerful "political machine" (Anderson 2021, 174). On the other side of modernity—and in the COVID present perhaps more than ever—predictive models and epidemiological projections tend to occupy the widening gap between experience

---

[1] Berlant also uses the expressions: "genre of the stretched out-present" and "genre of the emerging event." See Berlant (2011, 5).

and expectation. They solicit narrative interventions: stories whose role it is to entertain and edify (from *The Decameron* to 10 seasons of *The Walking Dead*), to anticipate (as in simulation scenarios run by security preparedness agencies), or as in *Driftwood* and Bauhin's chronicle to register the meaninglessness of a tick or and wolf bite as a social event. Amidst recent calls to "model responsibly" (Satelli et al. 2020, 484) and redefine modeling as a social activity, *Epidemiological Realism* ventured another model in which close readers, not unlike epidemiologists, relate observations to conjectures, generate exemplarity out of scatterings, and attend to emerging temporal relations that may or may not go anywhere. For what is epidemiology, if not a mode of being on the lookout for signs in a state of incipiency and a training in attentiveness tending to the agency of elusive patterns?

Bibliography

Abbott Pandemic Defense Coalition. 2023. The Virus Hunt: USA. https://www.youtube.com/watch?v=t686Kibr1-A. Accessed on June 28, 2024.

Altschuler, Sari. 2017. The Gothic Origins of Global Health. *American Literature* 89 (3): 557–590.

———. 2021. After the Outbreak. Narrative, Infrastructure, and Pandemic Time. *Resilience* 8 (3): 126–155.

Anderson, Benedict. 1983. *Imagined Communities: Reflections on the Origin and Spread of Nationalism*. London: Verso.

Anderson, Warwick. 2021. The Model Crisis, or How to Have Critical Promiscuity in the Time of Covid-19. *Social Studies of Science* 51 (2): 167–188.

Appadurai, Arjun. 1996. *Modernity at Large: The Cultural Dimension of Globalization*. Minneapolis: University of Minnesota Press.

Ariès, Philippe. 1971. *Essais sur l'histoire de la mort en occident du moyen âge à nos jours*. Paris: Seuil.

Barker, Sheila. 2004. Poussin, Plague and Early Modern Medicine. *The Art Bulletin* 86 (4): 659–689.

Barthes, Roland. 1968. L'effet de réel. *Communications* 11: 84–89.

———. 1975. *The Pleasure of the Text*, trans. Richard Miller. New York: Hill and Wang.

———. 1993. "La Peste": Annales d'une épidémie ou roman de la solitude? In *Oeuvres Complètes*, t. 1 (1942–1965), 452–456. Paris: Seuil.

Bauhin, Jean. 1591. *Histoire notable de la rage des loups, advenue l'an M.D.XC*. Foillet.

Belling, Catherine. 2009. Overwhelming the Medium: Fiction and the Trauma of Pandemic Influenza in 1918. *Literature and Medicine* 28 (1): 55–81.

© The Editor(s) (if applicable) and The Author(s), under exclusive license to Springer Nature Switzerland AG 2024
V. Bruyere, *Epidemiological Realism*, Palgrave Studies in Literature, Science and Medicine, https://doi.org/10.1007/978-3-031-68517-0

———. 2014. Andromeda's Futures: A Story of Humanities, Technology, Science, and Art. In *Health Humanities Reader*, ed. Therese Jones, Delese Wear, Lester D. Friedman, and Kathleen Pachucki, 409–418. New Brunswick: Rutgers University Press.

Belting, Hans. 2014. The Coat of Arms and the Portrait: Two Media of the Body. In *An Anthropology of Images: Picture, Medium, Body*, trans. Thomas Dunlap, 62–83. Princeton: Princeton University Press.

Benton, Adia. 2020. Border Promiscuity, Illicit Intimacies, and Origin Stories: Or What *Contagion*'s Bookends Tell Us About New Infectious Diseases and a Racialized Geography of Blame. Somatosphere. http://somatosphere.net/for umpost/border-promiscuity-racialized-blame/. Accessed on June 26, 2024.

Berlant, Lauren. 2011. *Cruel Optimism*. Durham: Duke University Press.

———. 2022. *On the Inconvenience of Other People*. Durham: Duke University Press.

Berlant, Lauren, and Jay Prosser. 2011. Life Writing and Intimate Publics: A Conversation with Lauren Berlant. *Biography* 34 (1): 180–187.

Borchers, Andrea T., Christopher Chang, and Eric Gershwin. 2017. Mold and Human Health: A Reality Check. *Clinical Review of Allergy and Immunology* 52 (3): 305–322.

Bourdeau, Loïc. 2022. Robin Campillo's *120 Battements Par Minute*, or When the Dust Unsettles. *Intertexts* 26 (1–2): 111–127.

Boyle, Danny, director. 2002. *28 Days Later*. Fox Searchlight Pictures. 113 minutes.

Bratton, Benjamin. 2021. *The Revenge of the Real: Politics for a Post-pandemic World*. London: Verso.

Braun, Bruce. 2008. Thinking the City Through SARS: Bodies, Topologies, Politics. In *Networked Disease: Emerging Infections in the Global City*, ed. Harris Ali and Roger Keil, 250–266. Oxford: Wiley-Blackwell.

Caduff, Carlo. 2014. Sick Weather Ahead: Data-Mining, Crowd-Sourcing and White Noise. *Cambridge Anthropology* 32 (1): 32–46.

———. 2015. *The Pandemic Perhaps: Dramatic Events in a Public Culture of Danger*. Berkeley: University of California Press.

Campillo, Robin, director. 2017. *120 Beats Per Minute*. Memento Films. 140 minutes.

Campillo, Robin, and Didier Péron. 2017. Chaque action d'Act Up était déjà enrobée par la fiction. *Libération*, August 20.

Camus, Albert. 1991. *The Plague*, trans. Stuart Gilbert. New York: Vintage Books.

Canguilhem, Georges. 1991. *The Normal and the Pathological*, trans. Carolyn R. Fawcett. Brooklyn: Zone Books.

Cazdyn, Eric. 2012. *The Already Dead. The New Time of Politics, Culture, and Illness*. Durham: Duke University Press.

CDC Public Health 101. 2024. Introduction to Epidemiology. https://www.cdc.gov/training-publichealth101/php/training/introduction-to-epidemiology.html. Accessed on June 28, 2024.

Chambers, Tod. 2017. Against "We", or an Argument for a Pluralistic Definition of Personhood in Bioethics. *AJOB Neuroscience* 8 (3): 173–174.

Chémery, Valentin, Juliette Farjat, Stéphane Gérard, Aude Lalande, Laure Vermeersch, and Sophie Wahnich. 2018. Mémoire vive. Politique et sida dans *120 Battements par minute*. Entretien avec Philippe Mangeot. *Vacarme* (82): 104–115.

Colebrook, Claire. 2020. A Remarkable Brain. *Identities: Journal for Politics, Gender and Culture*. https://identitiesjournal.edu.mk/index.php/IJPGC/announcement/view/39. Accessed on June 18, 2024.

Conis, Elena. 2015. *Vaccine Nation: America Changing Relationship with Immunization*. Chicago: Chicago University Press.

Cooter, Roger. 2013. *Writing History in the Age of Biomedicine*. New Haven: Yale University Press.

Cronon, William. 2011. Foreword: The Pain of a Poisoned World. In *Toxic Archipelago: A History of Industrial Disease in Japan*, ed. Brett Walker, ix–xii. Seattle: University of Washington Press.

Crosby, Alfred. 1972. Conquistador y Pestilencia. In *The Columbian Exchange: Biological and Cultural Consequences of 1492*, 35–60. Westport: Greenwood Publishing.

Crutch, Sebastian J., Ron Isaacs, and Martin N. Rossor. 2001. Some Workmen Can Blame Their Tools: Artistic Change in an Individual with Alzheimer's Disease. *Lancet* 357: 2129–2133.

De Man, Paul. 1973. Semiology and Rhetoric. *Diacritics* 3 (3): 27–33.

———. 1984. *The Rhetoric of Romanticism*. New York: Columbia University Press.

de Maupassant, Guy. 1888. *Pierre et Jean*. Paris: Ollendorff.

———. 1922. *Sur l'eau. The Magic Couch. And Other Stories*, trans. Albert McMaster London: Classic Publishing Company.

———. 1986. *Le Horla*, ed. André Fermigier. Paris: Folio Classique.

———. 2003. The Entity. In *The Necklace and Other Tales*, trans. Joachim Neugroschel. New York: The New York Library.

Derrida, Jacques. 2009. *The Beast and the Sovereign*, vol. 1, ed. Michel Lisse, Marie-Louise Malet, and Ginette Michaud, trans. Geoffrey Bennington. Chicago: University of Chicago Press.

Devere, Ronald. 2015. Still Alice: A Wonderful Movie with Superb Acting That Sends the Wrong Clinical Message. *Practical Neurology*: 43–44.

Dixon, Deborah P., and John Paul Jones. 2014. The Tactile Topologies of *Contagion*. *Transactions of the Institute of British Geographers* 40 (2): 223–234.

Doane, Mary Anne. 1980. The Voice in the Cinema: The Articulation of Body and Space. *Yale French Studies* 60: 33–50.

Duden, Barbara. 1993. *Disembodying Women: Perspectives on Pregnancy and the Unborn*, trans. Lee Hoinacki. Cambridge, MA: Harvard University Press.

Dwan, Allan, director. 1947. *Driftwood*. Republic Pictures. 88 minutes.

Felski, Rita. 2011. Context Stinks! *New Literary History* 42 (4): 573–591.

Flanagan, Mike, director. 2018. *The Haunting of Hill House*. Flanagan Film-Amblin Television-Paramount Television. 10 episodes, 42–71 minutes.

Fossier, Arnaud. 2011. La contagion des péchés (xie–xiiie siècle). Aux origines canoniques du biopouvoir. *Tracées* 21: 23–39.

Foucault, Michel. 1977. *Discipline and Punish*, trans. Alan Sheridan. New York: Random House.

———. 1994. La poussière et le nuage (1980). In *Dits et Ecrits*, t. IV, ed. Daniel Defert and François Ewald. Paris: Gallimard.

Franklin, Sarah. 2007. *Dolly Mixtures: The Remaking of Genealogy*. Durham: Duke University Press.

Furetière, Antoine. 1690. Dictionnaire universel. http://www.furetière.eu. Accessed on June 28, 2024.

Girard, René. 1974. The Plague in Literature and Myth. *Texas Studies in Literature and Language* 15 (5): 833–850.

Glatzer, Richard, and Wash Westmoreland, directors. 2014. *Still Alice*. Sony Pictures Classics. 101 minutes.

Gomel, Elana. 2000. The Plague of Utopias: Pestilence and the Apocalyptic Body. *Twentieth Century Literature* 46 (4): 405–433.

Ghosh, Amitav. 2016. *The Great Derangement: Climate Change and the Unthinkable*. Chicago: Chicago University Press.

Halbwachs, Maurice. 1913. *La théorie de l'homme moyen. Essai sur Quételet et la statistique morale*. Paris: Félix Alcan.

Hall, Stuart. 1992. Cultural Studies and Its Theoretical Legacies. In *Cultural Studies*, ed. Lawrence Grossberg, Cary Nelson, and Paula Treichler, 277–294. New York and London: Routledge.

Hamberger, Eric Stephen, and Bonnie Halpern-Felsher. 2020. Vaping in Adolescents: Epidemiology and Respiratory Harm. *Current Opinion in Pediatrics* 32 (3): 378–383.

Hartman, Geoffrey H. 1995. On Traumatic Knowledge and Literary Studies. *New Literary History* 26 (3): 537–563.

Hausner, Jessica, director. 2019. *Little Joe*. BFI Distribution. 105 minutes.

Haynes, Todd. director. 1995. *Safe*. Sony Pictures Classics. 119 minutes.

Hayot, Eric. 2009. *The Hypothetical Mandarin: Sympathy, Modernity, and Chinese Pain*. Oxford: Oxford University Press.

———. 2011. On Literary Worlds. *Modern Language Quarterly* 72 (2): 129–161.

———. 2012. *On Literary Worlds*. Oxford: Oxford University Press.

Hill, Richard E., Jr. 2005. Center for Veterinary Biologics Notice No. 05-23. United States Department of Agriculture. Animal and Plant Health Inspection Service—Center for Veterinary Biologics, December 8.

Huet, Marie-Hélène. 2012. *The Culture of Disaster*. Chicago: Chicago University Press.

Jain, S. Lochlann. 2013. *Malignant: How Cancer Becomes Us*. Berkeley: University of California Press.

James, Natalie Erika, director. 2020. *Relic*. Stan-IFC Midnight. 89 minutes.

Jameson, Fredric. 1985. The Realist Floor-Plan. In *On Signs*, ed. Marshall Blonsky, 373–383. Baltimore: Johns Hopkins University Press.

———. 2003. The End of Temporality. *Critical Inquiry* 29 (4): 695–718.

———. 2010. Realism and Utopia in *The Wire*. *Criticism* 52 (3–4): 359–372.

———. 2015. *The Antinomies of Realism*. London: Verso.

Keck, Frédéric. 2010. *Un monde grippé*. Paris: Flammarion.

———. 2014. From Purgatory to Sentinel: Form/Event in the Field of Zoonoses. *Cambridge Anthropology* 32 (1): 47–61.

———. 2015. L'alarme d'Antigone. *Terrain* 64: 3–19.

———. 2019. A Genealogy of Animal Diseases and Social Anthropology (1870–2000). *Medical Anthropology Quarterly* 33 (1): 24–41.

———. 2020. *Signaux d'alerte: Contagion virale, justice sociale, crises environnementales*. Paris: Desclée de Brouwer.

Keck, Frédéric, and Christos Lynteris. 2018. Zoonosis: Prospects and Challenges for Medical Anthropology. *Medical Anthropology Theory* 5 (3): 1–14.

Keetley, Dawn. 2021. Black Mold, White Extinction: *I Am the Pretty Thing That Lives in the House*, *The Haunting of Hill House*, "Gray Matter," and H. P. Lovecraft's "The Shunned House." In *Haunted Nature: Entanglements of the Human and the Nonhuman*, ed. Sladja Blazan, 43–66. Cham: Palgrave Macmillan.

Kenner, Alison. 2018. *Breathtaking: Asthma Care in a Time of Climate Change*. Minneapolis: University of Minnesota Press.

King, Nicholas B. 2004. The Scale Politics of Emerging Diseases. *Osiris* 19: 62–76.

Kornbluh, Anna. 2015. The Realist Blueprint. *The Henry James Review* 36 (3): 199–211.

Koselleck, Reinhart. 2004. *Futures Past: On the Semantics of Historical Time*, trans. Keith Tribe. New York: Columbia University Press.

Kupferschmidt, Kai. 2012. Attack of the Clones. *Science* 337 (6095): 636–638.

Lacan, Jacques. 2017. Conférence de Louvain. *La Cause Du Désir* 96: 7–30.

Lachenal, Guillaume, and Gaetan Thomas. 2020. Epidemics Have Lost the Plot. *Bulletin of the History of Medicine* 94: 670–689.

Landecker, Hannah. 2013. When the Control Becomes the Experiment. *Limn* 3. http://limn.it/when-the-control-becomes-the-experiment/. Accessed on June 28, 2024.

Latour, Bruno. 2005. *Reassembling the Social: An Introduction to Actor-Network Theory*. Oxford: Oxford Univ. Press.

Law, John, and Annemarie Mol. 2011. Veterinary Realities: What Is Foot and Mouth Disease? *Sociologia Ruralis* 5 (1): 1–16.

Leiris, Michel. 1930. L'Homme et son intérieur. *Documents* 5: 261–266.

Léonard, Jacques. 1980. L'historien et le philosophe. In *L'Impossible Prison: Recherches sur le système pénitentiaire au XIXe siècle*, ed. Michelle Perrot, 9–28. Paris: Seuil.

Lipkin, Ian. 2011. Helping Hollywood Create and Battle a Pandemic. *Science* 333 (6047): 1219.

Lock, Margaret. 2013. *The Alzheimer Conundrum: Entanglements of Dementia and Aging*. Princeton: Princeton University Press.

Love, Heather. 2016. Small Change: Realism, Immanence, and the Politics of the Micro. *Modern Language Quarterly* 77 (3): 419–445.

Lukács, Georg. 1971. Narrate or Describe? In *Writer and Critic, and Other Essays*, ed. and trans. Arthur Kahn, 110–148. London: Merlin Press.

Lynteris, Christos. 2020a. Didactic Historicism and the Historical Consciousness of Epidemics. *Somatosphere*. http://somatosphere.net/forumpost/didactic-historicism-historical-consciousness-epidemics/. Accessed on June 2024.

———. 2020b. *Human Extinction and the Pandemic Imaginary*. New York: Routledge.

Ma, Ling. 2018. *Severance: A Novel*. New York: Farrar, Straus and Giroux.

Mader, Mary Beth. 2012. *Sleights of Reason: Norm, Bisexuality, Development*. Albany: State University of New York Press.

Marin, Louis. 1989. *Food for Thought*, trans. Mette Hjort. Baltimore: Johns Hopkins University Press.

Massumi, Brian. 2010. The Future Birth of the Affective Fact. The Political Ontology of Threat. In *The Affect Theory Reader*, ed. Melissa Gregg, Gregory J. Seigworth, 52–70. Durham: Duke University Press.

Mills, Jennifer. 2018. "A Concoction of Bitterness and Sweetness": An Interview with Ling Ma. *The Lifted Brow* 45, October 2.

Montaigne, Michel. 1958. *The Complete Essays of Montaigne*, ed. and trans. Donald Frame. Stanford: Stanford University Press.

Mortimer, Philip P. 2003. Five Postulates for Resolving Outbreaks of Infectious Disease. *Journal of Medical Microbiology* 52: 447–451.

Murphy, Michelle. 2006. *Sick Building Syndrome and the Problem of Uncertainty. Environmental Politics, Technoscience, and Women Workers*. Durham: Duke University Press.

Murphy, Monica, and Bill Wasik. 2012. Summer of Rage: Rabies Surge in Some States Might Be Due to Heat. *Wired*, July 26.

Nersessian, Anahid. 2020. *The Calamity Form: On Poetry and Social Life.* Chicago: Chicago University Press.

One Health High-Level Expert Panel (OHHLEP). 2022. One Health: A New Definition for a Sustainable and Healthy Future. *PLOS Pathogens* 18 (6). https://doi.org/10.1371/journal.ppat.1010537. Accessed on June 28, 2024.

Ostherr, Kirsten. 2005. *Cinematic Prophylaxis: Globalization and Contagion in the Discourse of World Health.* Durham: Duke University Press.

Panofsky, Erwin. 1955. The History of Art as a Humanistic Discipline. In *Meaning in the Visual Arts. Papers in and on Art History*, 1–25. Garden City: Anchor Books.

Pata, John, director. 2023. *Black Mold.* Head Trauma Productions. 92 minutes.

Petersen, Wolfgang, director. 1995. *Outbreak.* Warner Bros. 128 minutes.

Post, S.G. 1995. Alzheimer Disease and the "Then" Self. *Kennedy Institute of Ethics Journal.* 5 (4): 307–321.

Povinelli, Elizabeth. 2006. *The Empire of Love: Toward a Theory of Intimacy, Genealogy, and Carnality.* Durham, NC: Duke University Press.

Preciado, Paul, B. 2020. Learning from the Virus. *Artforum* 58 (9). https://www.artforum.com/features/learning-from-the-virus-247388/. Accessed on June 18, 2024.

Raaf, Sabrina. 2006. Breath Cultures. In *Going Aerial: Air, Art, Architecture*, ed. Monika Bakke, 34–35. Maastricht: Jan van Eyck Academie.

Rancière, Jacques. 2017a. *Les Bords de la fiction.* Paris: Seuil.

———. 2017b. Madame Aubain's Barometer. In *The Lost Thread: The Democracy of Modern Fiction*, trans. Steven Corcoran, 3–26. London: Bloomsbury.

Raza Kolb, Anjuli Fatima. 2020. *Epidemic Empire: Colonialism, Contagion, and Terror, 1817–2020.* Chicago: Chicago University Press.

Reid, Roddey. 1998. UnSafe at Any Distance: Todd Haynes' Visual Culture of Health and Risk. *Film Quarterly* 51 (3): 32–44.

Rosenberg, Charles. 1973. *The Cholera Years: The United States in 1832, 1849, and 1866.* Chicago: University of Chicago Press.

———. 1989. What Is an Epidemic? AIDS in Historical Perspective. *Daedalus* 118 (2): 1–17.

Roy, Arundhati. 2020. The Pandemic Is a Portal. *Financial Times*, April 3.

Sade, Donatien. 1973. *Voyage d'Italie, ou Dissertations critiques, historiques, politiques et philosophiques sur les villes de Florence, Rome et Naples (1775–1776).* In *Œuvres complètes*, vol. XVI. Paris: Tête de Feuilles.

Saffire, Linda, and Adam Schlesinger, directors. 2016. *Restless Creature: Wendy Whelan.* Abramorama. 90 minutes.

Satelli, Andreas, et al. 2020. Five Ways to Ensure That Models Serve Society: A Manifesto. *Nature* 582: 482–484.

Sedgwick, Eve. 2003. Paranoid Reading and Reparative Reading; or, You're So *Paranoid*, You Probably Think This Essay Is About You. In *Touching Feeling: Affect, Pedagogy, Performativity*, 123–151. Durham: Duke University Press.

Serres, Michel. 1994. *Atlas*. Paris: Juillard.

Silva, Cristobal. 2011. *Miraculous Plagues: An Epidemiology of Early New England Narrative*. Oxford: Oxford University Press.

Sirucek, Stefan. 2014. Ancient 'Giant Virus' Revived From Siberian Permafrost. *National Geographic*, March 3.

Soderbergh, Steven, director. 2011. *Contagion*. Warner Bros. Pictures. 106 minutes.

Sodikoff, Genese. 2016. Mad and Mythical Dogs. 3 Quarks Daily. https://3quarksdaily.com/3quarksdaily/2016/10/mad-and-mythical-dogs.html. Accessed on June 26, 2024.

———. 2017. Multispecies Epidemiology and the Viral Subject. In *Routledge Companion to the Environmental Humanities*, ed. Ursula Heise, Jon Christensen, and Michelle Niemann, 112–119. London: Routledge.

Squier, Susan. 2004. *Liminal Lives: Imagining the Human at the Frontiers of Biomedicine*. Durham: Duke University Press.

Steedman, Carolyn. 2002. *Dust: The Archive and Cultural History*. New Brunswick, NJ: Rutgers University Press.

Stoichita, Victor. 1997. *The Self-Aware Image: An Insight into Early Modern Meta-Painting*. New York: Cambridge University Press.

Strauss, Jonathan. 2012. *Human Remains: Medicine, Death, and Desire in Nineteenth-Century Paris*. New York: Fordham University Press.

Van Haver, Luc, and Xavier Reyé, directors. 2015. *Quand C'est?* Mosaert-Benuts. 3:15 minutes.

Wald, Priscilla. 2008. *Contagious: Cultures, Carriers, and the Outbreak Narrative*. Durham: Duke University Press.

Watney, Simon. 1987. The Spectacle of AIDS. *October* 43: 71–86.

Weber, Samuel. 2022. *Preexisting Conditions: Recounting the Plague*. Brooklyn: Zone Books.

Weisman, Alan. 2007. *The World Without Us*. New York: Picador-Thomas Dunne Books.

Woodward, Kathleen. 1999. Statistical Panic. *differences* 11 (2): 177–203.

Woolf, Virginia. 1926. On Being Ill. *The New Criterion* 4 (1): 32–45.

Yazell, Bryan, and Hsuan L. Hsu. 2020. Naturalist Compulsion, and the Time-Loop Zombie. *CR: The New Centennial Review* 20 (3): 23–46.

Zhang, Dora. 2020. Staying Alive. *Post45*. https://post45.org/2020/10/staying-alive/. Accessed on June 18, 2024.

Zola, Émile. 1894. *Germinal*, trans. Havelock Ellis. London: Dent and Sons Ltd.

SPRINGER NATURE

GPSR Compliance

The European Union's (EU) General Product Safety Regulation (GPSR) is a set of rules that requires consumer products to be safe and our obligations to ensure this.

If you have any concerns about our products, you can contact us on ProductSafety@springernature.com

In case Publisher is established outside the EU, the EU authorized representative is:

Springer Nature Customer Service Center GmbH
Europaplatz 3
69115 Heidelberg, Germany